The Congestive Heart Failure Mastery Bible: Your Blueprint For Complete Congestive Heart Failure Management

Dr. Ankita Kashyap and Prof. Krishna N. Sharma

Published by Virtued Press, 2023.

THE CONGESTIVE HEART FAILURE MASTERY BIBLE: YOUR BLUEPRINT FOR COMPLETE CONGESTIVE HEART FAILURE MANAGEMENT

First edition. November 20, 2023.

ISBN: 979-8215552001

Written by Dr. Ankita Kashyap and Prof. Krishna N. Sharma.

Table of Contents

.... 1
Introduction 2
Understanding Congestive Heart Failure 5
Medical Insights 6
Symptoms Decoded 9
Living With CHF 12
Real Patient Stories 15
Family and Caregiver Perspective 18
Mental Health and CHF 21
Holistic Understanding 24
Medical Management of CHF 27
Diagnostic Procedures 28
Medication Management 31
Surgical Interventions 34
Rehabilitation and Recovery 37
Emerging Treatments 40
Palliative Care 43
Clinical Trials and Research 46
Lifestyle Modifications and Self-Care 48
Dietary Guidelines 49
Exercise and Physical Activity 51
Stress Management Techniques 55
Sleep Hygiene and CHF 58
Smoking Cessation and CHF 61
Alcohol and CHF 64
Mind-Body Connection 66
Emotional Wellness and Support 69
Coping With Diagnosis 70
Family Dynamics and Relationships 73
Peer Support and Community 76
Therapeutic Outlets 79

Seeking Professional Help 82
Spirituality and Faith 85
Resilience and Hope 88
Supportive Care and Practical Strategies 91
Care Coordination and Advocacy 92
Financial Resources and Assistance 95
Home Care and Assistance 97
Transportation and Mobility 100
Nutritional Support and Meal Planning 102
Legal and Ethical Considerations 105
Patient Empowerment and Self-Advocacy 108
Holistic Approaches to CHF Management 111
Herbal Remedies and Supplements 112
Acupuncture and Traditional Chinese Medicine 115
Ayurveda and Holistic Wellness 118
Energy Healing and Reiki 121
Mindfulness and Meditation 124
Aromatherapy and Relaxation Techniques 127
Integrative Medicine and Collaborative Care 130

DISCLAIMER

The information provided in this book is intended for general informational purposes only. The content is not meant to substitute professional medical advice, diagnosis, or treatment. Always consult with a qualified healthcare provider before making any changes to your diabetes management plan or healthcare regimen.

While every effort has been made to ensure the accuracy and completeness of the information presented, the author and publisher do not assume any responsibility for errors, omissions, or potential misinterpretations of the content. Individual responses to diabetes management strategies may vary, and what works for one person might not be suitable for another.

The book does not endorse any specific medical treatments, products, or services. Readers are encouraged to seek guidance from their healthcare providers to determine the most appropriate approaches for their unique medical conditions and needs.

Any external links or resources provided in the book are for convenience and informational purposes only. The author and publisher do not have control over the content or availability of these external sources and do not endorse or guarantee the accuracy of such information.

Readers are advised to exercise caution and use their judgment when applying the information provided in this book to their own situations. The author and publisher disclaim any liability for any direct, indirect, consequential, or other damages arising from the use of this book and its content.

By reading and using this book, readers acknowledge and accept the limitations and inherent risks associated with implementing the strategies, recommendations, and information contained herein. It is always recommended to consult a qualified healthcare professional for personalized medical advice and care.

Introduction

Currently, I am composing the preface for "The Congestive Heart Failure Mastery Bible: Your Comprehensive Guide to Congestive Heart Failure Treatment." The chance to share with you the conclusion of a trip that has influenced not only my career path but also my personal beliefs humbles me. As a physician and health and wellness coach, I have devoted my professional life to advancing holistic medicine and wellness, viewing my patients as unique persons in need of thorough, caring treatment rather than just cases. This book, a work of love that pulls from both the heights and the depths of my experience to provide you with a guide on how to manage congestive heart failure with dignity, fortitude, and empowerment, is a monument to that dedication.

My foray into the field of healthcare and wellness was not only a career move, but also a profoundly personal voyage that sparked a passion for me to promote the holistic health of people with long-term illnesses. True healing, in my opinion, goes beyond the purview of conventional medicine, based on both my personal experiences and those of the people I have had the honour to treat. It requires a balanced fusion of medical expertise, humane treatment, and a deep understanding of the numerous variables affecting a person's health and wellbeing.

I have developed a distinct viewpoint that serves as the foundation for this book by drawing on my experiences, successes, and significant obstacles that I have faced along the road. The pages you are holding in your hands bear witness to the never-ending search for new information, the steadfast dedication to evidence-based practise, and the passionate belief in the transforming potential of holistic medicine. This book is not just the result of my experience; it is a gift from the heart that will help you and countless others who are attempting to navigate the maze that is congestive heart failure.

I was well aware of the responsibility that comes with managing a disease as intricate and varied as congestive heart failure when I set out on this project. I engaged in extensive study, reading reputable scientific papers, consulting reliable medical publications, and condensing a plethora of information into a clear, understandable storey in order to piece together this thorough guide. Every word and every sentence is rife with the wisdom that can only be obtained from painstaking research and a deep commitment to helping those in need.

Through the course of my career, I have had the privilege of earning honours and recognition that, in addition to being medals of honour, also act as lights of hope, confirming my thought leadership and groundbreaking contributions to the field of holistic healthcare. Rather than lying idly on the shelves of my memory, these honours bear witness to the steadfast dedication to excellence that forms the foundation of this book. They provide witness to the faith that my mentors and colleagues have in me, and in me, as I provide you with an insight into the potentially revolutionary nature of integrative heart failure care.

But underneath the surface of honours and recognition from the industry is a very intimate bond with the topic at hand. Through the tears, the victories, and the undying perseverance of the patients I have had the honour to treat, a bond has been created. The heart of this book is the tapestry of empathy and understanding that their experiences, hardships, and unyielding spirit have weaved within me. This is more than just a technical guide; it's an ode to the human spirit's tenacity, a celebration of the victories and the unshakable bravery of people who face congestive heart failure head-on.

As you begin your journey through the pages of "The Congestive Heart Failure Mastery Bible," I cordially ask you to become a part of an elite group of enlightened individuals, a communion of spirits and minds bound by a common goal of resilience and empowerment. This book is more than just an accumulation of information; it's a key to a world where congestive heart failure, empowerment, and resilience come together to show the way forward. It is an invitation to adopt a new healthcare paradigm that recognises the transformative power of holistic management techniques and moves beyond the limitations of traditional approaches.

You will find a painstakingly designed road map for resolutely and gracefully negotiating the intricacies of congestive heart failure in the pages that follow. I have made an effort to equip you with practical solutions, adaptable programmes, and self-help techniques that address the particular needs of each person facing this disease by combining a harmonic blend of medical knowledge and holistic perspectives. This book is more than just an informational resource; it is a ray of hope and proof of the life-changing potential that is inside each and every one of us, just waiting to be discovered and developed.

I offer you my hand, my heart, and my steadfast dedication to assisting you in finding a path of empowerment and fortitude in the face of congestive heart failure as we set out on this life-changing adventure together. Together, let's embrace the knowledge contained in these pages and allow it to be your road map to total congestive heart failure management.

Understanding Congestive Heart Failure

Medical Insights

Chapter Subtitle: Unraveling the Intricacies of Congestive Heart Failure

My dear reader,

Let's take a moment to explore the fundamentals of congestive heart failure (CHF) before we set out on this adventure to comprehend and master its intricacies. The heart contains a symphony of physiological mechanisms that, when disturbed, can result in the unrelenting chaos of congestive heart failure. The heart is the chamber where life's beat is arranged. This subchapter will delve into the intricate details of congestive heart failure (CHF), including its severe effects on heart function, the critical role blood circulation plays, and the long-term effects it has on important organs.

Let's start this journey by losing ourselves in the heart's symphony, an organ that constantly regulates the ups and downs of existence. The fundamental cause of CHF is a discordant note that echoes across the cardiovascular system, disrupting the otherwise harmonious symphony. Our main goal is to shed light on the physiological processes that underlie this illness, with the goal of deciphering the mysterious dance of the heart and its effects on the complex network of our body's operations.

We make the following claim: CHF is a severe disruption that affects the entire body rather than just a cardiac condition. In order to verify this claim, let us first examine the workings of the heart, which is the hub of this never-ending maelstrom. The amazing muscle known as the heart beats with all the vitality of a living being, pumping blood full of oxygen to every part of the body. However, when CHF weighs on it, this essential organ fails to do its function as it tries to keep the blood flowing in a steady pace.

This is where we find our first piece of evidence: the heart's impaired function in CHF. Imagine the heart as a brave conductor, directing blood through the complex system of vessels in a harmonious manner. This conductor falters in CHF, the heart's chambers unable to pump blood efficiently, the symphony halting. The consequences of this compromised function are felt throughout the body, affecting key organs like the liver, kidneys, and lungs.

Examining this data in greater detail reveals the significant consequences of impaired blood circulation in congestive heart failure. Think of the circulatory system as a major thoroughfare, with blood travelling along its lanes to carry vital oxygen and nutrients. But when CHF is present, this highway gets clogged, making it difficult for the body's cells and tissues to receive the life-sustaining nutrition they need. This causes the body's essential organs to go without the food they so sorely need, which has a series of upsetting effects.

We now come across contradicting evidence as we work our way through the maze of CHF, which calls into question our first assertion. There are others who contend that congestive heart failure (CHF) only affects the heart and its chambers. To refute this claim, nevertheless, we need to shed light on the extensive effects of CHF on the body's essential organs. The systemic aspect of CHF is demonstrated by the liver's congestion, the kidneys' struggle with reduced blood flow, the lungs' difficulty eliminating extra fluid from the body, and the liver itself.

We respond to this counter-evidence by restating our claim: CHF is a condition that does, in fact, extend beyond the walls of the heart, looming large over the complex network of body functions. Allow us to present more proof in favour of this position: the significant effect that CHF has on the body's metabolic functions. Consider the body's metabolism as a symphony of chemical interactions, a delicate ballet necessary to keep life alive. This dance is upset in the presence of CHF, which sets off a series of imbalances that put additional strain on the heart and other essential organs.

Finally, we reiterate our position with steadfast conviction: CHF is a severe disruption that affects every part of the body, not only the heart. By figuring out the physiological principles underlying this illness, we can better understand the extensive effects it has on essential organs and body processes. Let us not waver in our pursuit of comprehension as we descend more into CHF, for it is only by knowledge and discernment can we open the door to victory over this unrelenting foe.

With unyielding determination,
Dr. Ankita Kashyap

Symptoms Decoded

Greetings, cherished readers, and welcome to an enlightening voyage through the complex network of symptoms that unveil the murmurs of silent congestive heart failure. This subsection will delve into the mysterious language of the body, interpreting the different cues and indicators that require our scrutiny. Imagine yourself as a detective as we set out on our exploration, piercing the surface to reveal the secrets that are concealed within. Let's explore the diverse range of symptoms, each of which tells a different tale of the heart's fight.

Envision a busy clinic that is brimming with vitality. Through its corridors pass patients from various walks of life, each with a distinct tale imprinted in the lines of their faces. The symphony of symptoms plays out here in this dramatic environment, with each note bearing the stories of those looking for comfort and understanding. Whispers and murmurs, waiting to be understood, are the language of the heart speaking among the din of conversations and the steady pounding of medical equipment.

Introducing Sarah, a lively fifty-year-old whose laughter used to fill every space she went into. She is now so exhausted that even the act of walking up a flight of stairs makes her gasp for air. James, the stoic gentleman seated across the room, has a rhythmic swelling in his legs and ankles that breaks up his once-steady walk. These people, and a plethora of others, are the protagonists in the storey of congestive heart failure; everyone has a distinct storey that demands understanding.

Sometimes the heart, our faithful friend, fails to perform its function properly because of congestive heart failure. The difficult part is figuring out the small cues that this important organ gives, which are sometimes covered up as symptoms that seem harmless. Breathlessness, exhaustion, edoema, and erratic heartbeats are just a few of the numerous indicators that beg us to solve their riddles. Because of the intricacy of these symptoms, diagnosing their importance and assisting our patients in their healing requires both a sharp eye and a loving heart.

Congestive heart failure is managed differently in the context of holistic healthcare and wellbeing than it is in conventional medicine. It includes a patchwork of coping mechanisms, individualised meal and nutrition planning, psychiatric counselling, and lifestyle adjustments. Every aspect of our strategy is designed to address the complex nature of the symptoms, with the goal of promoting long-term wellbeing in addition to reducing their immediate impact. By adopting this all-encompassing strategy, we enable our patients to take an active role in their quest for heart health.

We see firsthand the transformative power of comprehending and treating the variety of symptoms associated with congestive heart failure as we proceed down this path of compassionate care and holistic recovery. Sarah's chuckle, muffled by exhaustion, reverberates through her life's hallways. James moves with fresh purpose and energy after being freed from the weight of swelling. The benefits of our method go beyond the simple relief of symptoms; they include a renewed sense of energy and happiness, which enhances the lives of people we assist.

We see a mirror reflecting the complex interactions between the mind, body, and spirit in the tapestry of symptoms. It makes us consider the deep relationships that exist between emotional health and outward appearances. The lessons learned from these encounters force us to recognise the constraints and uncertainties that come with the healing process while also serving as a reminder of the transforming power of a comprehensive approach.

Imagine a diagram that illustrates how symptoms are related to one another, like a tiny net that the heart whispers in. Each strand stands for a unique symptom that is closely connected to the others to create a cohesive picture of comprehension and support.

Understanding the symptoms is a microcosm of our larger goal, which is to provide light on the route to total care of congestive heart failure. Weaving a storey of empowerment and resiliency as we decipher the language of the heart promotes a profound comprehension of the body's signals and the significant influence of holistic wellbeing. In the pursuit of vibrant health, this journey is about more than just understanding symptoms; it's about accepting the profound interdependence of mind, body, and spirit.

What if we saw symptoms as profound messages from the body, asking us to listen to it and respond with empathy and compassion, rather than just as physical signs of a disease? The patchwork of symptoms may hold the key to life-changing understanding and treatment. Let's take a moment as we carry on our investigation to consider the tales that our symptoms convey and the lessons they might impart to those who are open to hearing them.

We shall explore the complex dance of symptoms and treatments in greater detail in the pages that follow, providing guidance toward total control over the treatment of congestive heart failure. Come along on this fascinating journey with me as we explore the mysteries of the heart and adopt a holistic philosophy that goes beyond the confines of conventional medicine. Let's set out on a life-changing path to healthy heart health and wellness together.

Living With CHF

We must manage not just the medical complexities of managing Congestive Heart Failure (CHF), but also the day-to-day adaptations and challenges that those who live with this condition must make. Living with congestive heart failure (CHF) involves several facets, such as maintaining physical and mental well-being and dietary restrictions. Resilience, flexibility, and a wholistic attitude to wellbeing are necessary on this journey.

Let's begin by setting the scenario. Imagine a life in which each breath serves as a constant reminder of the careful balancing act between symptom management and experiencing life to the fullest. For those who have congestive heart failure (CHF), even seemingly easy actions might seem like enormous undertakings. Every facet of daily life is impacted by CHF, from the ordinary to the remarkable, creating a special fabric of struggles and victories.

The main problem is that people with CHF have to manage their daily lives very carefully in order to lessen the effects of the ailment. The complicated nature of having CHF is exacerbated by the unpredictable nature of symptoms, the necessity of rigorous adherence to treatment regimens, and the possibility of exacerbations. Maintaining a sense of normalcy while adjusting to the condition's constant realities is a delicate dance.

There are serious repercussions if the difficulties of having CHF are not addressed. People may suffer from a reduction in their general quality of life, more hospital stays, and an elevated risk of complications in the absence of aggressive management. The constant watchfulness needed to control CHF can be taxing on mental health and social connections, which can lead to a decline in emotional well-being.

So, what is the solution? It entails adopting a holistic perspective that includes food adjustments, self-care methods, lifestyle adjustments, and procedures for mental well-being. Despite the difficulties presented by CHF, people can actively manage their disease and work toward a full life by incorporating these components into their daily lives.

The first step in putting these methods into practise is to have a thorough grasp of the particular requirements and constraints that each person with CHF faces. It is essential to take a customised approach that is based on the unique circumstances and preferences of each individual. This could entail working with a multidisciplinary team of specialists, comprising dietitians, mental health specialists, and healthcare professionals, to develop a comprehensive care plan that takes into account the psychological, emotional, and physical components of having congestive heart failure.

Previous results, which show better symptom control, fewer hospitalizations, and an improved quality of life for those with CHF, have proven the effectiveness of this strategy. Through the integration of dietary adjustments, self-care practises, and lifestyle alterations, people have demonstrated increased resilience and optimism in the face of CHF's problems.

Although this all-encompassing strategy is the cornerstone of managing CHF, it's important to recognise that there are other options. Every person's experience with CHF is different, so what works for one person might not work for another. People with CHF can benefit from additional levels of support and empowerment when they explore alternative therapies and complementary strategies.

Living with congestive heart failure is like setting out on a journey with an ever-changing horizon. Every day brings with it fresh successes and obstacles, necessitating flexibility and fortitude. It's about accepting life to the fullest even with CHF; it's not just about controlling symptoms.

It is important to keep in mind that every person has the ability to influence their own experience as we negotiate the challenges of living with congestive heart failure. People can build a life that goes above the limitations put in place by CHF with the correct help, direction, and all-encompassing commitment to wellbeing. Although the path requires unyielding resolve, it also offers the possibility of resilience, hope, and the joy of experiencing life to the fullest, despite the difficulties presented by CHF.

Real Patient Stories

Numerous tales are told in the medical field both in the homes and hearts of patients, as well as within the walls of hospitals. These tales are more than just anecdotes; they are vivid, breathing examples of the human spirit's resiliency and victory. I have had the honour of witnessing these stories of bravery and tenacity as a medical practitioner and health and wellness coach, particularly in the context of congestive heart failure. Everybody has a different journey, one that is full of obstacles, successes, and the moving dance between optimism and despair. I would like to share with you a few of these true patient stories that have had a profound impact on my comprehension of this intricate and multidimensional illness.

Picture a calm hospital room that is softly lit by the evening sun coming through the windows. A background of muted urgency is created by the quiet whispers of the medical professionals and the unceasing beeping of the monitors, serving as a constant reminder of life's fragility. The lives of those suffering from congestive heart failure play out in this calm yet intense environment, each with its own beat and rhythm.

One such person is Maria, a lively and enthusiastic lady in her late 60s whose enthusiasm for life was evident in all she said. Even as she navigated the maze of symptoms and obstacles presented by congestive heart failure, her eyes shone with warmth and knowledge. Michael, a stoic and resolute man in his mid-50s, is another important character. His strong commitment to his family is only surpassed by his unwavering desire to face his health issue head-on. Many others, like these people, turned into the heroes of their own tales, with congestive heart failure acting as an unexpected enemy.

Congestive heart failure, a disorder that threatened to overwhelm their lives with its crippling symptoms and unpredictable prognosis, was the main obstacle that these people had to face. Their days were shadowed by the weight of exhaustion, the smothering grip of dyspnea, and the constant worry of flare-ups, making them wonder that they could lead happy and full lives.

Given these enormous obstacles, our strategy went well beyond the traditional boundaries of medical care. We explored the complex web of holistic health care, which includes dietary and lifestyle adjustments, customised counselling, psychology-related procedures, self-help methods, coping mechanisms, and alternative and complementary forms of self-care. Every person's path was meticulously customised to meet their own requirements and circumstances, giving them the ability to take back control of their health and wellbeing.

This all-encompassing approach produced results that were truly amazing. After being bound by exhaustion, Maria started taking leisurely strolls in the park under the sun, her laughter infectious and upbeat. Now, his eyes full of immense delight, Michael, who had battled the crushing grip of breathlessness, rejoiced in the simple joy of playing catch with his grandkids. These were not merely anecdotal; rather, they were validated by observable enhancements in their clinical parameters, highlighting the significant influence of integrative healthcare on the management of congestive heart failure.

These patient anecdotes serve as a reminder of the efficaciousness of a multifaceted approach to healthcare. We were able to awaken each person's latent potential and improve their life beyond the limitations of their diagnosis by accepting the interdependence of the mind, body, and spirit. But there were many unknowns and difficulties along the way, which is why we had to keep improving and changing our methods to better meet the requirements of the people we were looking after.

The graphic depictions that encapsulate the core of these patient stories—the transformational journey, the interaction between vulnerability and resilience, and the significant effects of managing congestive heart failure holistically—can be found in the pages that follow.

These patient tales are threads woven into the greater narrative of managing congestive heart failure, not stand-alone narratives. They act as moving reminders of the human condition, which is characterised by perseverance, bravery, and the unwavering quest of a life well lived. They highlight how essential holistic healthcare is to changing the paradigm of managing chronic diseases and provide a model for all-encompassing, compassionate care.

I ask you to consider the following as you go through 'The Congestive Heart Failure Mastery Bible: Your Blueprint for Complete Congestive Heart Failure Management'. What hidden reserves of fortitude and resiliency are there in every person just waiting to be discovered thanks to holistic healthcare's healing abilities? This question invites us to explore farther into the core of the human experience, where inspiring tales of hope and triumph are waiting to be spoken, much like a guiding star in the night sky.

Family and Caregiver Perspective

The effects of congestive heart failure (CHF) go well beyond the person who has been diagnosed, as is clear when we examine the complex web of care around this illness. In order to provide CHF patients with constant support, family members and caregivers must navigate a difficult dance that involves emotional, physical, and practical obstacles. Together, we can unravel this delicate tapestry and shed light on the critical role that families and caregivers play in providing patients with CHF with comprehensive treatment.

Imagine a family gathering in a warmly lit living room to talk about the most recent advancements in their loved one's fight against CHF. There's a tangible will to overcome the obstacles ahead mixed with a distinct weight of worry in the air. The effect of CHF permeates every discussion and choice made here, in the soft embrace of familial love.

The patients with congestive heart failure (CHF) and the unsung heroes who support them are the main characters in this storey. These heroes are the family members and caregivers; they all have a special tale to tell and a common goal of lifting their loved ones' spirits. Their vocations and backgrounds are as different as they are, but what unites them is their unrelenting commitment to lessening the hardships experienced by CHF.

The main obstacle is that CHF is a complex illness that impacts not just the patient's physical health but also the mental well-being of everyone in the patient's care system. Families and caregivers are faced with a multitude of challenges, ranging from comprehending the complexities of prescription schedules to managing the emotional upheaval that results from watching a loved one struggle with a chronic illness.

Empowerment turns into a lighthouse that leads caregivers and families through the maze of CHF. In my experience as a health and wellness coach, providing families with information, tools, and coping mechanisms has a profoundly positive effect. Our goal is to strengthen the network of support that surrounds people with CHF by providing individualised lifestyle modifications, holistic counselling, and self-care strategies that promote resilience and optimism in the face of hardship.

The results of this method penetrate not just clinical measures but also the core structure of family relationships. I have seen a daughter who was initially intimidated by her father's complicated treatment plan grow into a strong supporter of her father's health. Mutual understanding and group resilience strengthen the familial link while sharing the load of caring and relieving the strain of uncertainty.

This path is not without difficulties, though. Careful consideration is necessary due to the psychological effects on caregivers, the pressure on family dynamics, and the practical challenges of juggling caregiving and personal obligations. By recognising these intricacies, we can adapt our strategy and guarantee that caregivers and families get the comprehensive assistance they need to successfully negotiate the maze of CHF.

Consider a graph that shows the emotional arc of a caregiver, with the peaks representing resilience and the valleys representing fatigue. This graphic illustration serves as a moving reminder of the emotional rollercoaster that people who are responsible for providing care for CHF patients go through.

A microcosm of the comprehensive care paradigm—which is essential to managing congestive heart failure—is the viewpoint of the family and caregiver. Similar to how the complex workings of the heart work together to maintain life, the patients' support system needs to work together to foster understanding, hope, and unwavering support. Through highlighting the critical role that families and caregivers play, we shed light on the connection between individual well-being and group resilience while dealing with CHF.

Let's consider the following as we begin this examination of the complex tapestry that is CHF: How can we strengthen the safety net of understanding, information, and resilience that surrounds CHF patients? This inquiry challenges us to go farther, peel back the layers of caregiver and family interactions, and come away with a comprehensive grasp of our shared path toward holistic CHF treatment.

Mental Health and CHF

Title: Taking Care of the Heart Inside: Maintaining Mental Well-Being Despite Congestive Heart Failure

Greetings, readers, and welcome to the complex dance of the heart and mind in the context of congestive heart failure (CHF). As we explore the complex and numerous aspects of comprehensive CHF management, it is critical to draw attention to the often-underappreciated but enormously influential field of mental health. We will explore the resilient spirit and coping strategies that are the cornerstone of holistic well-being in this subchapter, which will take us beyond the physical symptoms of CHF. Let's examine the maze of feelings, steer clear of the resilient waves, and show the way toward mental toughness when dealing with CHF.

Picture a calm, well-lit space with the soft hum of medical equipment and the calming presence of kind caregivers. Here, in the heart clinic, we see people attempting to make their way through the winding hallways of congestive heart failure. Their tales are as varied as the hues of a sunset, each filled with a special mixture of successes and setbacks. The storey of managing CHF is shaped by the complex interactions between physical and mental health that take place in this hallowed area.

Meet Mrs. Patel, a vibrant matriarch who, in spite of her serious CHF diagnosis, has a laugh that reverberates throughout the clinic's hallways. Her unflinching fortitude and will to appreciate life's small pleasures are examples of the human spirit's tenacity in the face of hardship. Beside her is Dr. Singh, a sympathetic cardiologist who recognises that comprehensive therapy goes beyond prescription drugs. When it comes to managing CHF, they represent the mutually beneficial interaction between physical and mental health.

For patients and their loved ones, receiving a CHF diagnosis frequently signals a drastic change in direction in life. The constant ns combined with the fear of dying can have a ne's mental state. The inherent resilience that each ..ı be threatened by overwhelming feelings of ...y, melancholy, and impending loss. Providing for mental health in the middle of CHF's turmoil becomes a critical task that calls for a multimodal strategy based on compassion and understanding.

The mental health canvas in the sanctuary of comprehensive CHF management is painted in a multitude of hues, each of which stands for a different aspect of coping and resilience. Patients are given a safe space to express their hopes and worries through individualised counselling, which promotes empowerment in the face of vulnerability. Additionally, the combination of breathing exercises, meditation, and mindfulness practises is like a balm for the spirit; it gives everyone a fresh sense of inner peace. In addition, the acceptance of peer networks and support groups weaves a tapestry of common experiences and fosters a feeling of solidarity in the face of hardship.

The rewards for our efforts to support mental health in the face of CHF are abundant. Patients such as Mrs. Patel, who was formerly caught in the maze of hopelessness, are now positively charged and resilient. The reduction of anxiety and despair, the development of coping mechanisms, and the reinforcement of mental resilience serve as evidence of the transformative potential of comprehensive care. Empirical evidence also reveals a decrease in readmissions to hospitals and an improvement in quality of life, highlighting the mutually beneficial interaction between mental and physical health.

Whenever we traverse the fabric of mental health in the context of CHF, it is critical to recognise the possible objections and difficulties. Seeking help can be hampered by the stigma associated with mental health in some cultural contexts, thus a nuanced and culturally sensitive approach is required. Furthermore, a deliberate effort must be made to break down the silos that frequently divide physical and psychological treatment in order to incorporate mental health support into the framework of CHF management. Through the promotion of a smooth and continuous healthcare system, we may create a storey of comprehensive health that goes beyond traditional thinking.

Picture a graphic mosaic in which the colours of resiliency, the shapes of coping, and the subtle qualities of mindfulness are all woven together. These visual tools provide a moving picture of hope in the face of hardship and stand as a tribute to the transformational power of fostering mental well-being amidst CHF.

The domain of mental health becomes an integral part of CHF management, permeating all facets of intervention. We can transcend the limitations of physical ailments and create a path toward ultimate well-being by tending to the heart within. The human spirit's resiliency emerges in the sanctuary of mental toughness, brilliantly illuminating the path of managing CHF.

While we enjoy the symphony of health amid CHF, let us consider: In what ways may we continue to sow the seeds of mental toughness, creating a fabric of health that reaches beyond the confines of illness? Come along with me as we solve the mystery of mental toughness and show you how to fully conquer CHF.

The throbbing pulse of resilience reverberates through the halls of CHF management in the complex dance of heart and mind, illuminating the path to holistic well-being. Together, let's set out on a journey that goes beyond the boundaries of suffering, embracing the transformational potential of mental toughness and tending to the inner heart.

Holistic Understanding

Adopting a holistic perspective of this complicated illness is essential to managing congestive heart failure effectively. We're taking care of a complete person, with complex relationships spanning the mind, body, and spirit, rather than merely treating a physical illness. This method explores areas beyond traditional medicine, including lifestyle changes, complementary and alternative medicines, and the significant influence of general health on illness management. As we explore the connections between many facets of health and wellness in the context of congestive heart failure, let's go on a voyage of holistic understanding.

That being said, what does it mean to treat congestive heart failure holistically? It involves more than just taking care of the condition's physical symptoms and symptoms. Rather, it's about understanding the complex relationship between health and wellness and how each component of our lives affects our overall wellbeing.

To put it simply, holistic understanding is combining traditional medical procedures with complementary and alternative methods to treat the mental, social, and spiritual aspects of the patient in addition to the physical symptoms of congestive heart failure. It highlights how managing chronic illnesses like congestive heart failure and preserving general health depend on the interconnection of the mind, body, and spirit.

The term "holistic understanding" refers to a broad range of factors that influence a person's general state of wellbeing. This covers dietary and exercise changes, stress reduction methods, social support, emotional and psychological support, and the use of complementary and alternative therapies. We can develop a more thorough and individualised strategy to managing congestive heart failure by addressing these crucial components.

A holistic perspective on congestive heart failure reveals that the illness is interconnected with the patient's overall life. Instead, it is intricately linked to many facets of their lives, such as their relationships, routines, emotional and mental health, and general sense of fulfilment and purpose. Comprehending the wider context around congestive heart failure enables us to customise our treatment to the particular requirements and situations of every person.

Think about the effects of managing congestive heart failure with stress-relieving techniques like yoga or meditation. These methods may have a beneficial impact on physiological functions like lowering blood pressure and enhancing cardiovascular health, in addition to fostering relaxation and mental health. By incorporating these techniques, we can improve the general health of people who have congestive heart failure.

A prevalent misunderstanding regarding holistic methods is that they are in some way antagonistic to traditional medical interventions. The truth is that holistic knowledge improves and supplements conventional medical treatments, providing a more thorough and individualised method of treating congestive heart failure. To maximise the general well-being of people with this illness, the best aspects of both worlds should be integrated rather than one over the other.

We will examine the significant effects of lifestyle changes, the integration of complementary and alternative therapies, and the critical role that emotional and psychological support play in illness management as we delve deeper into the holistic understanding of congestive heart failure. Together, we'll reveal how different facets of health and wellbeing are interconnected, creating a clear picture of a holistic knowledge that goes beyond the confines of conventional medical paradigms.

As we navigate the difficulties of congestive heart failure, we'll weave together conventional treatment and holistic techniques to create a rich tapestry of well-being. Join us on this transforming journey through the pages that follow. So let us go on this journey of holistic knowledge, recognising the unity of the body, mind, and spirit as we steer toward total care of congestive heart failure.

Medical Management of CHF

Diagnostic Procedures

Greetings from the wonderful world of congestive heart failure diagnostic techniques, dear reader. As diligent investigators gather evidence to solve a riddling case, so too do we, as medical professionals, utilise a variety of diagnostic techniques and tests to solve the riddles of congestive heart failure and direct our patients toward the best possible care and well-being.

Even with its fearsome nature, congestive heart failure is not immune to our investigative skills. This chapter will take us on a tour of the diagnostic environment, examining the instruments and methods that enable us to reveal the complex mechanisms of the heart and its environment. Every diagnostic examination, from the soft beeps of an echocardiogram to the steady pulse of stress testing, provides a crucial hint towards unlocking the mystery of congestive heart failure.

The central hypothesis of our investigation is that, through gaining a thorough understanding of the diagnostic processes involved in congestive heart failure, we can enable patients and healthcare professionals to make well-informed decisions and steer towards integrated care and enhanced quality of life.

The echocardiography, a non-invasive, illuminating procedure that uses sound waves to capture the heart in motion, is the cornerstone of our diagnostic arsenal. The structure, operation, and integrity of the heart's pumping mechanism are all clearly shown by this dynamic image. We uncover a tapestry of information as we explore the complexities of the echocardiography, from the subtleties of valve operation to the subtle ebb and flow of blood within the chambers.

Think of the echocardiography as a skilled painter who skillfully captures the sound waves on a canvas to represent the heart's symphony. The echoing heart reveals the thickness of its walls, the size of its chambers, and the force of its contractions with every beat. We can identify any structural anomalies, such as dilated chambers or compromised valve function, through this complex dance of sound and visuals, providing insight into the underlying causes of congestive heart failure.

However, we come against the echocardiogram's limitations in our quest for clarity. Although it provides a clear picture of the structure and operation of the heart, it might not always identify the underlying causes of heart failure, such as coronary artery disease or minute electrical irregularities. To properly understand the complex nature of congestive heart failure, we thus need to augment our diagnostic toolkit with other resources.

In order to tackle these intricacies, we resort to the domain of blood tests, where an array of biomarkers subtly conveys stories of heart strain, inflammation, and compromised performance. Like a storyteller's quill, the insignificant blood sample tells the storey of the heart's struggles and leads us to a better comprehension of the underlying pathophysiology. Furthermore, several tests function as sentinels, indicating the existence of cardiac distress and offering vital information regarding the severity and prognosis of congestive heart failure. Examples of these tests are B-type natriuretic peptide (BNP) and troponin levels.

Stress tests become an increasingly useful diagnostic tool as we broaden our scope because they mimic the heart's response to effort and reveal latent symptoms of ischemia or reduced pumping capacity. Moreover, sophisticated imaging methods, such as cardiac MRIs and CT scans, provide a broad perspective of the heart's structure and reveal minute details that are missed by traditional imaging modalities.

Each thread in the tapestry of congestive heart failure diagnostic methods weaves together to create a complete picture that sheds light on the subtleties of the situation and directs us toward customised therapeutic approaches. Accepting the complexity of diagnostic testing gives us the ability to deconstruct congestive heart failure, enabling both patients and healthcare providers to take a more comprehensive approach to health and vibrantly live.

Medication Management

Welcome to the realm of congestive heart failure (CHF) medication management, where compassion and science come together to offer a thorough approach to treating this complicated illness. As we explore the field of pharmacological therapies, it is imperative to comprehend the critical role that drugs play in reducing symptoms, improving cardiac function, and preventing adverse events. Our goal is to enable people with CHF to take advantage of the promise of holistic wellness and lead happy, full lives through the thoughtful integration of pharmaceutical therapy.

The problem of congestive heart failure is complex and requires a complex approach to treatment. Fatigue, dyspnea, and fluid retention are just a few of the symptoms that result from the body's critical organs and tissues being denied oxygen and key nutrients by the heart's inability to pump blood efficiently. When these symptoms come together, it can drastically lower someone's quality of life and make daily tasks difficult. Medication management plays a pivotal role in the overall treatment of congestive heart failure (CHF) in this regard.

The main difficulty in treating CHF is striking a careful balance between treating the underlying causes of heart failure and its symptoms. To create a regimen that meets the individual needs of every patient, we must sort through the complex web of medications, each with its own mode of action and possible adverse effects. Moreover, the ever-changing character of CHF demands ongoing monitoring and pharmacological regimen modifications to accommodate the patient's changing requirements.

Inadequate medication management in patients with congestive heart failure (CHF) can have far-reaching effects on all facets of their lives. Unmanaged symptoms can cause crippling bouts of dyspnea, frequent hospital stays, and a reduced ability to carry out everyday tasks. In addition, neglecting to enhance cardiac performance and slow down the advancement of heart failure may result in an increased chance of potentially fatal consequences, so sustaining a vicious cycle of doubt and diminished health.

We support a thorough and customised approach to drug management to address these issues. By combining the most recent evidence-based recommendations with a thorough comprehension of each patient's particular situation, we are able to create a customised drug schedule that aims to reduce symptoms, improve heart function, and halt the advancement of CHF.

The successful execution of our medication management approach is contingent upon a thorough evaluation of the patient's clinical profile, encompassing their symptoms, co-occurring conditions, and drug tolerance. To provide the best possible symptom alleviation and improve cardiac function, we start by titrating the right doses of important drugs, such as beta-blockers, diuretics, and angiotensin-converting enzyme (ACE) inhibitors. Our goal is to achieve a delicate balance that supports both stability and vitality by continuously monitoring the patient's response and modifying the regimen as needed.

We also stress the significance of patient empowerment and education as we negotiate the terrain of medication management. Our patients take an active role in their own care, and we provide the information and resources they require to understand their prescription schedule, identify any possible adverse effects, and follow the recommended course of action. By using this cooperative method, we develop a partnership based on mutual respect and trust, as well as a sense of agency and understanding that goes beyond the simple use of pharmaceuticals.

The amazing changes we see in our patients are a testament to the success of our drug management strategy. With a drug regimen customised to meet their specific needs, people who previously struggled with the debilitating grip of persistent symptoms experience relief and a revitalised sense of energy. Not only does optimising cardiac function improve their quality of life on a daily basis, but it also acts as a ray of hope, giving them courage and strength to face the challenges of chronic heart failure.

We acknowledge the importance of supplementary modalities that might enhance the advantages of pharmacological therapies, even though medication management remains a fundamental component of the all-encompassing therapy of CHF. The range of possible supplementary techniques is extensive and includes anything from dietary and lifestyle changes to the incorporation of complementary therapies like yoga and acupuncture. We want to promote a collaborative approach that goes beyond the confines of conventional drug management by adopting a holistic framework that considers all aspects of a patient's health.

To sum up, the practise of managing medication for congestive heart failure involves more than just writing prescriptions; it involves a deep dedication to promoting each patient's health and resiliency. Equipped with the most recent developments in medical science and a humane comprehension of the human condition, we are ready to set the path for a bright and promising future in CHF management as we set off on our adventure.

Surgical Interventions

We approach a critical turning point in the treatment of congestive heart failure (CHF) where conventional medical instruments and state-of-the-art surgical procedures collide. Imagine the following scenario: a patient, Mr. Smith, is confronted with the difficult task of having severe CHF. It's time to investigate the world of surgical possibilities since his heart, the very engine of life, is fighting an uphill battle. Explore the world of ventricular assist devices, heart transplants, and other cutting-edge medical techniques, all of which offer the prospect of a longer and better life.

Our key characters in this unfolding storey are the devoted medical staff and, of course, the strong patients themselves. The protagonist of this storey is Mr. Smith, a living example of the resilience of the human spirit. His tale serves as a powerful reminder of the human ability to persevere in the face of great adversity because it is one of bravery and steadfast resolve.

The task at hand is evident: guiding patients through the perilous reaches of severe CHF while providing a route to recovery and vigour. This is no easy task, as the consequences are really high. The choices made here will determine how Mr. Smith's destiny unfolds as he dances a precarious dance between life and death.

We are taking a comprehensive approach to this enormous task, leveraging the technological marvels of today along with the knowledge of surgical pioneers. For patients like Mr. Smith, a heart transplant—which formerly seemed like something out of science fiction—has turned into a real lifesaver. Ventricular assist devices, a technical marvel that offers both short-term and long-term relief for failing hearts, are a monument to human ingenuity. In the face of insurmountable odds, these cutting-edge medical techniques provide a glimmer of hope and the possibility of a new lease on life.

Let's now concentrate on the outcomes of these surgical procedures. The results are practically miraculous. Patients who had previously faced the threat of death are now allowed a fresh lease on life, with their hearts pounding with increased vitality. The data is self-explanatory, presenting a clear picture of surviving and prospering following these medical miracles. Every successful surgery is a monument to the unwavering spirit of the human heart, both literally and figuratively, and a victory of human persistence and medical innovation.

A deep sense of amazement descends upon us as we pause to consider and evaluate these remarkable results. The lessons learned from these situations are both humble and deep. They serve as a constant reminder of the incredible capacity for human invention and the remarkably resilient nature of the human spirit. However, we also have to admit that there are drawbacks and difficulties with these surgical procedures. This seemingly wonderful scene is shadowed by sombre realities such as the limitations of medical resources, the complexity of organ donation, and ethical problems.

Visual aids can be really helpful in our understanding process because they provide concrete examples of these intricate medical procedures. The reader has a deeper understanding of these complex ideas by witnessing the deft choreography of expert hands and the complicated ballet of medical equipment, which puts these ideas in a relatable and understandable context.

However, we must not lose sight of the bigger storey that is being told here. The surgical procedures that we have looked at are essential components of the larger picture of managing CHF rather than stand-alone cures. They stand for the forefront of a patient-centered, holistic approach to healthcare that skillfully combines the wonders of contemporary medicine with the fundamental principles of holistic wellness.

As we shift our focus, one question remains unanswered: How can society as a whole keep pushing the envelope of medical innovation while guaranteeing that these life-saving therapies are accessible to all? It's an issue that needs to be addressed collectively because it forces us to think about the moral, societal, and financial implications of sophisticated surgical procedures for congestive heart failure.

In conclusion, the surgical procedures performed on CHF patients are a monument to the amazing advancements in contemporary medicine, providing new life and hope to those who previously faced overwhelming challenges. While we should be happy for these accomplishments, we also need to proceed cautiously and consider the wider ramifications and difficulties that come with these novel techniques.

Surgical interventions provide a bright point of hope in the larger picture of CHF management, showing the way to a day when lives can be rejuvenated and hearts can be healed. And may us, walking on the edge of what was once thought unattainable, bring with us the profound lessons and insights learned from the amazing world of surgical procedures as we continue our journey through the pages of "The Congestive Heart Failure Mastery Bible."

Rehabilitation and Recovery

: Nurturing the Heart Back to Health

It becomes essential to stop and consider the path to recovery as we navigate the complex web of congestive heart failure. The road to healing and rehabilitation is not just a set of exercises to follow and food changes to make; it is a complete metamorphosis, a complex dance involving the body, mind, and soul. This subchapter delves into the fundamental significance of cardiac rehabilitation programmes, examining their critical role in helping persons navigating the maze of congestive heart failure to restore physical function, improve quality of life, and foster long-term recovery.

Imagine a symphony, where every instrument plays in unison with the others to create a soul-stirring combination of melody. Our bodies are intricate orchestrations as well, with the heart acting as the conductor and setting the pace for life. But when the heart's song becomes an unharmonious cacophony, when the symphony breaks, it becomes necessary to embark on the healing road. The path to recovery in the case of congestive heart failure is fraught with obstacles, yet hope is seen when viewed through the lens of holistic rehabilitation.

The main concern here is the severe effects of congestive heart failure on a person's physical and mental health. The toll that sickness takes on one's capacity to perform daily tasks, the never-ending cycle of exhaustion and dyspnea, and the psychological strain of adjusting to a life changed by disease. These are the obstacles that must be overcome in order to have a full and active life, and doing so requires steadfast resolve.

In the event that these issues are not resolved, dire repercussions are imminent. Every day that goes by is evidence of one's life ebbing away, happiness eroding, and hope gradually fading. If treatment is not received, the effects of congestive heart failure can affect all facets of life, including the most basic pleasures.

The light of hope shines on the path of rehabilitation and recovery, pointing us in the direction of cardiac rehabilitation programmes' transformational power. These programmes are healing havens that provide a variety of methods for body and spirit renewal as well as reviving an enthusiasm for life.

The road to recovery opens up little by little. It starts with an extensive examination, a mosaic of health assessments and one-on-one conversations that reveal the particular requirements of every person. After that, a customised programme is developed that includes physical activity, dietary advice, stress reduction methods, and mental health assistance. Each component works in unison to create a unified approach that tackles the complex nature of congestive heart failure.

The success of cardiac rehabilitation programmes is audible and overwhelming. Previous results attest to the recovery of bodily functions, the reduction of symptoms, and the resuscitation of hope. The projections shine brightly as we look to the future, showing us glimpses of lives regained, hearts thumping with new vitality, and people embracing a life redefined by resiliency and vibrancy.

Heart rehabilitation programmes are a powerful ally on the road to recovery, but it's important to recognise that there are other options that can work in concert with this strategy. Every option—from cutting-edge medical procedures to integrative therapies—presents a potential thread in the rehabilitation process. But the combination of these strategies, entwined with the ideas of comprehensive care, is what has the capacity to foster significant change.

Let us go out on this road with steadfast commitment, embracing the transformational potential of holistic treatment, as we navigate the maze of rehabilitation and recovery. Every stride toward recovery becomes evidence of the human spirit's tenacity, a healing and hope-filled symphony that resonates with the prospect of a full and active life. Restoring the heart to health is within our reach as we set out on a path lit by the light of possibilities. Let's set out on this journey of rejuvenation together, led by the life-changing heart rehabilitation programmes.

Emerging Treatments

Greetings from a world of possibility and inventiveness, where science and hope mingle. We are about to set off on a journey that has the potential to change people's lives and entirely rewrite the history of this complicated illness as we explore the most recent developments in medical therapy for congestive heart failure.

Imagine a society in which the unyielding will to heal is combined with the unrelenting quest of knowledge. In this context, the future of congestive heart failure treatment is being woven together by innovative research and medical advancements. With the ultimate goal of improving the quality of life for those affected by this ailment, we see the emergence of novel therapies and the development of time-honored methods within this dynamic environment.

The dedicated researchers, the creative physicians, and the brave patients who take part in clinical trials are at the core of these developments, working together to push the limits of what is feasible in the treatment of congestive heart failure. Their combined commitment ignites the advancement engine and pushes us to explore new avenues for care and treatment.

The difficulty stems from Congestive Heart Failure's complex nature, which necessitates a multimodal care strategy. Every facet poses a different challenge to conquer, ranging from the careful balancing act on fluid retention to the constant demand on the heart muscle. Even while conventional therapies have been very helpful, there is still a relentless search for more focused, efficient interventions that can actually alter the course of this illness.

Now let's talk about new medicines, which are changing the landscape of congestive heart failure care like a symphony of creativity. The array of therapy options is growing, ranging from cutting-edge surgical treatments that provide new hope for people in need of interventions to innovative drugs created to target particular pathways implicated in the evolution of the condition. In addition, the incorporation of holistic therapies, lifestyle adjustments, and customised treatment plans gives the approach additional depth and nuance, acknowledging the body, mind, and spirit's interconnectedness in the quest for holistic wellness.

The results are quite telling and provide a clear picture of the revolutionary potential of these new therapies. Patients who previously struggled with incessant symptoms get relief, having their vitality returned and their spirits raised. These stories are supported by the data, which shows improvements in important cardiac function indicators and patient-reported outcomes that highlight the real effects of these creative strategies. Congestive heart failure may not be a death sentence in the future—rather, it will be only one chapter in a greater tale of resiliency and rejuvenation—as the body of evidence grows.

However, as we go through this progressive landscape, we need to stop and consider the lessons these developments teach us. We have to continue to be diligent in our inspection, realising that although innovation has great potential, it also necessitates thoughtful deliberation and continuous assessment. What drawbacks and dangers can these novel treatments have? How can we strike the careful balance between welcoming advancement and protecting against unintended consequences? These are the kinds of inquiries that highlight the accountability that accompanies breaking new ground in the medical field.

Visual aids provide windows into the world of new treatments within the pages of this subchapter, revealing the complex systems at work as well as the palpable effects of these interventions. The intricacy of scientific ideas is communicated through graphical representations and images, which also provide a visual foundation and entice the reader to go further into the world of innovation.

The storey of congestive heart failure is not separate; rather, it is deeply interwoven with the overall theme of holistic health and well-being. It personifies the philosophy of individualised, patient-centered care, in which the patient takes an active role in their own path to wellbeing rather than just receiving care. It emphasises how interdisciplinary collaboration may be transformative, combining medical knowledge, holistic approaches, and patient advocacy to produce a care plan that goes beyond established limits.

Let us consider the enormous significance of these achievements as we consider the panorama of developing therapeutics. How might they influence how congestive heart failure is managed in the future—not just in terms of medicine, but also in terms of the experiences of those who are impacted by the illness? How can we, as guardians of health and well-being, support and direct the development of these therapies? These are the inquiries that invite us to delve further into the game-changing potential of innovation in healthcare.

In the pages that follow, we'll take you on an engrossing voyage into the world of cutting-edge therapies, revealing the strands of advancement and opportunity that could completely alter the way congestive heart failure is managed. Come with me as we explore the centre of invention, where possibilities abound and hope finds a home.

Palliative Care

The goal of holistic wellbeing in the context of managing congestive heart failure (CHF) is a harmonious blend of empathy, comprehension, and unshakable commitment. As we explore the maze of CHF, we come across people whose lives are influenced not just by the physical limitations of their illness but also by the emotional upheaval that goes along with it. In this situation, palliative care plays a pivotal role in providing comfort, weaving a web of assistance that surpasses the confines of conventional medical treatment.

Imagine this: tired from the never-ending dance with CHF, the patient seeks not just a physical relief but also a haven where their concerns are allayed, their joy is restored, and their emotional well-being is fostered. Palliative care enters this scene as a lighthouse, illuminating the way towards holistic well-being with its roots firmly planted in the comprehensive care paradigm.

The main problem is not just the physical expression of CHF; rather, it's the intricate interactions between symptoms that affect every aspect of a patient's life. The mental and spiritual well-being of individuals coping with CHF is negatively impacted by the combination of exhaustion, dyspnea, and an unceasing rhythm of uncertainty.

In the absence of the gentle embrace of palliative care, the effects are severe and widespread. Untreated distress can have a profound emotional impact on a patient's life, upsetting the delicate equilibrium between hope and fortitude. The effects are felt far beyond the person, soaking into the fabric of social and familial ties and leaving a trail of unmet needs and unsaid grief in their wake.

Palliative care is a comprehensive approach that uses a soft touch to relieve the physical, emotional, and existential discomfort associated with chronic heart failure. It is a haven where patients' quality of life is greatly improved and their inner essence is fostered rather than just their symptoms being controlled.

Palliative care implementation is a delicate dance in which the evidence-based interventions and the compassion beat together. The first step is a comprehensive evaluation of the patient's needs, covering not only physical symptoms but also emotional health, spiritual comfort, and existential clarity. From there, a customised plan is developed that includes a variety of interventions, such as counselling, advanced care planning, and symptom management.

Palliative care's compassionate supervision fosters resilience and transformation, as demonstrated by the compelling data. In the midst of the storm, patients find comfort, regaining their happiness and welcoming life with fresh vitality. The emotional wounds start to heal and the weight of the symptoms lessens, opening the door to a life that is not just lived but treasured.

Palliative care, which recognises that the human experience cannot be reduced to just symptoms and diagnoses, acts as a guardian of holistic well-being while standard medical interventions focus on the clinical signs of CHF. For individuals making their way through the maze of CHF, it serves as a beacon of hope, a wellspring of consolation, and a cradle of comfort.

Symptom management stands out as the cornerstone of palliative care, providing relief from the constant weight of pain, exhaustion, and dyspnea. Imagine living a life in which every breath is a lovely song rather than a struggle, and every step is a graceful dance instead of a struggle. This is the promise of palliative care—a promise that reaches deep into the patient's experience and goes beyond the boundaries of conventional medical care.

Palliative care, however, offers more than just a break from physical suffering; it's a refuge for the spirit and a safe harbour for mental health. Patients can express their hopes, dreams, and anxieties in a safe environment here. It's a place where the turmoil of feelings finds meaning and where the burden of doubt is distributed. Counseling, psychological support, and compassionate listening help to relieve the emotional burden of CHF and restore resilience in the spirit.

Palliative care encompasses not just the physical and emotional aspects of a patient's journey, but also the existential and spiritual aspects as well. This is where advanced care planning becomes ingrained, giving patients the ability to direct their medical care in a way that is consistent with their values and beliefs. Here, the essence of life, the fabric of memories, and the legacy of love are combined to create a storey that knows no bounds.

Palliative care plays a critical role in improving the quality of life for individuals navigating the maze of congestive heart failure. This must be recognised as we negotiate the landscape of holistic care. Not only do palliative care services provide relief from symptoms, but they also serve as a spiritual retreat, a safe haven for emotional stability, and a place to find existential clarity. This, my dear friends, is the palliative care promise—a promise that reaches beyond the boundaries of conventional medical care and provides a glimmer of hope and healing to people impacted by the complications of congestive heart failure.

Clinical Trials and Research

It's critical to acknowledge the evolving character of medical science as we navigate the complex terrain of managing congestive heart failure (CHF). The advancement of CHF treatment is fueled by the unwavering search of information and innovation, which gives patients and medical professionals alike hope. This subchapter delves into the realm of clinical trials and research, where innovative ideas and unwavering dedication come together to forge new paths in the comprehension and treatment of congestive heart failure.

Picture yourself at the entrance of a busy lab, the sound of state-of-the-art machinery blending with the passionate energy of exploration. It's a thrilling field that constantly pushes the limits of medical understanding and offers hope and possibility to people facing the complications of congestive heart failure.

The researchers, doctors, and patients are the main players in this engrossing field; each one adds a distinct thread to the fabric of medical advancement. Their mutual dedication to solving the puzzle of CHF and creating novel solutions serves as the foundation for their cooperative efforts.

Our task is complex; it involves improving the efficacy of already available therapies, finding new therapeutic approaches, and improving the lives of those who are suffering with CHF. It is crucial to use research and clinical trials to overcome these challenges and improve the environment in which CHF patients are cared for.

Leading this effort are researchers who carefully plan and carry out clinical trials, each of which is evidence of the accuracy and commitment that guide their work. These studies provide as testing grounds for novel drugs, evaluations of various treatment approaches, and close examination of the effects of lifestyle modifications on the course of CHF.

The results of these arduous experiments and research projects are extensive, sparking advancements in healthcare that reverberate throughout the board. They produce priceless information that reveals the effectiveness of novel therapies, explains the complex network of systems underlying CHF, and opens up new possibilities for individualised care that goes beyond conventional boundaries.

Thinking back on the fabric created by research and clinical trials serves as a reminder of the underlying ambiguity surrounding medical inquiry. There are many detours on the way to knowledge, and although some of them lead to ground-breaking discoveries, others could take us in unexpected directions. However, it is via this process of trial and error that the advancement of medicine is assembled, with each piece adding to the overall picture of managing congestive heart failure.

Imagine a graph that shows how CHF treatment options have changed over time, highlighting the critical impact that research and clinical trials have played in changing the therapeutic environment.

The storey of the research and clinical trials blends in perfectly with the main idea of managing CHF holistically. It highlights how quickly medical knowledge is developing and how important it is to adopt cutting-edge tactics while never letting up in our quest for better patient care.

While navigating the maze-like passageways of medical research, consider this: What revolutionary discoveries are still to come that will allow CHF management to enter a new chapter? The answer lies, my dear readers, in the unknown, where curiosity is king and the adventurous spirit of exploration rules.

Lifestyle Modifications and Self-Care

Dietary Guidelines

Title: Taking Care of Your Heart: Nutritional Plans for Treating Congestive Heart Failure

Greetings from the beginning of your quest to overcome congestive heart failure, dear reader. As we set out on this life-changing journey together, it is critical to understand that wellbeing is rooted in the food we provide our bodies. Now, let's take a fascinating look at dietary recommendations that are especially designed to assist those who are suffering from congestive heart failure.

Our goal is very clear: we want to give you the information and know-how to optimise your diet in order to strengthen and nourish your heart. You will have a thorough understanding of the nutrient-dense foods, portion control, and fluid management that are essential for maintaining heart health by the end of this chapter.

All you need to go on this culinary journey with us is an open mind, an eagerness to try new things, and a desire to empower your body with the food you eat.

Let's pause to appreciate the stunning patchwork of dietary recommendations for the treatment of congestive heart failure. We'll delve into the complexities of nutrient-dense foods, examine the fine line between portion control, and traverse the sometimes disregarded field of fluid management.

1. Visualize your heart as a fragile flower growing in a garden that is fed by the varied hues and textures of foods high in nutrients. Enjoy the earthy deliciousness of entire grains, the crispness of leafy greens, the sweetness of berries, and the rainbow.

2. Consider portion control to be the conductor of a symphony, arranging nutrients and flavours in the ideal harmony. Accept the practise of mindful eating, appreciate each bite as though it were a work of art, and pay attention to your body's signals of fullness.

3. Visualize fluid management as the calm river's gradual rise and fall, providing your body with nourishment without becoming too much. Accept equilibrium, relish the crunch of unadulterated water, delight in the sweetness of fruit that is derived from water, and be aware of the concealed fluid content in some dishes.

As you venture forth, heed these nuggets of wisdom:

- Accept the idea of moderation and give yourself the odd treat while continuing to eat in a generally well-balanced manner.
- Plan your meals so that you may empower yourself to make wise selections and steer clear of snap judgments that might not be in your best interests.
- Consult a qualified dietitian for advice since they can offer individualised suggestions based on your unique dietary requirements and constraints.

An increased sense of vitality, a bounce in your step, and the soft hum of a healthy heart are signs that you are following a healthy diet.

If difficulties come up during your diet, keep in mind that failure does not equal setbacks. Rather, see them as chances for development and adjustment. Seek assistance from your medical team, and together, use resiliency and determination to successfully negotiate the maze of nutritional options.

As we come to the end of this insightful journey into nutritional recommendations, keep in mind that our health is a work in progress. Accept the practise of heart-nourishing, and delight in the harmonious blend of tastes and sensations that is holistic well-being.

May you travel a nutritional path that is informed, infused with delight, and directed by intention. We will feed our souls, strengthen our bodies, and relish the bounty of life's colourful palette together.

Exercise and Physical Activity

Greetings from the realm of exercise and physical activity, which can change lives, dear reader. We're going to go on an adventure to discover the potential of movement in the treatment of congestive heart failure in this chapter. We will examine the advantages of exercise, suitable training regimens, and crucial safety measures to maximise cardiovascular health as we go more into the topic.

This chapter's main goal is to identify safe and practical exercise recommendations for people with congestive heart failure. We'll uncover the ways that physical activity can improve general health and heart health.

It is imperative that you obtain your healthcare provider's approval before beginning any workout regimen. Along for the ride should also be adequate footwear and comfortable exercise clothes.

Let's start with a broad overview of the terrain surrounding physical activity and exercise. We'll discuss the main advantages, look at appropriate exercise techniques, and set the stage for a thorough method of incorporating physical activity into your daily routine.

The Benefits of Physical Activity:

Think of exercise as the heart's symphony—a beautiful tune that promotes stronger heart health, more endurance, and better circulation. Exercise strengthens your heart and improves your general health on a regular basis. Moving to the beat of your own rhythm can lower blood pressure, raise cholesterol, and give you a sense of vigour that spills over into every part of your life.

Appropriate Workout Routines:

As we go further into the world of exercise, we'll customise exercise plans to meet the particular requirements of individuals with CHF. We'll discuss a variety of workouts, from low-impact aerobics to gentle stretches, making sure that every motion you do is a step closer to reviving your heart and lifting your soul.

Precautions to Optimize Cardiovascular Health:

We'll navigate the oceans of exercise with care and caution, much like an experienced navigator plots a course with accuracy. We'll take the precautions and warnings seriously in order to keep your heart healthy, making sure that every action you take demonstrates your dedication to overall health.

Now, let's zoom in and dissect the components of safe and effective exercise for CHF patients.

Consultation with Healthcare Provider

It's important to speak with your healthcare professional before starting any fitness programme. They will evaluate your present state of health, offer tailored advice, and make sure your workout regimen suits your particular requirements.

Tailoring Exercise to Your Fitness Level

We'll personalise your training regimen to your present fitness level, just like a tailor makes a suit to fit flawlessly. We'll make sure your workout routine is both comfortable and effective, regardless of your level of experience.

Embracing Variety in Exercise Modalities

Variety is what makes life interesting, and the same is true when it comes to fitness. You will be able to embrace a spectrum of movement that nourishes your heart and spirit as we explore a tapestry of training methods, from mild yoga to aquatic workouts.

Monitoring Signs and Symptoms

We'll be alert for any indications or symptoms that may appear during activity, much like a sentinel. Through the recognition and response to your body's signals, we'll make sure that your fitness path is both safe and empowering.

As we continue our journey into the world of fitness, let's light the way with helpful advice and sobering recommendations.

Tip 1: Listen to Your Body

Your body whispers ideas that direct your exercise journey like a knowledgeable elder. Pay close attention to its cues, respecting its knowledge, and modifying your workout schedule as necessary.

Tip 2: Stay Hydrated

Your body benefits from being hydrated in the same way that a plant does when it is fed with water. Always have a bottle of water on available so that you can replenish your body's reservoir with each cool drink.

Warning 1: Avoid Overexertion

Excessive effort can be harmful, even though passion is commendable. Take it slow, enjoy every step, and refrain from physically demanding activities that could put strain on your heart.

Warning 2: Be Mindful of Weather Conditions

The aspects of nature might affect how you exercise. Be aware of high temperatures and adapt your workout schedule to suit the whims of the weather.

How can we tell whether our fitness routine is working? Now let's examine the signs of a job well done.

Indicator 1: Improved Stamina and Endurance

When you start exercising, you might experience a renewed sense of energy throughout your days. Your endurance and stamina will grow, giving you the energy to greet every day with fresh enthusiasm.

Indicator 2: Enhanced Cardiac Function

Your heart's rhythm will become stronger and more resilient as it echoes the symphony of movement. Exercise has the transforming power since your heart will function as a reflection of the loving care you've given it.

There may occasionally be difficulties while we negotiate the terrain of exercise. Let's arm ourselves with answers to typical issues that might come up.

Challenge 1: Difficulty Sustaining Motivation

Similar to a flickering flame, motivation can fluctuate. Take part in enjoyable activities, look for the companionship of encouraging peers, and commemorate each accomplishment to keep the spark of drive burning bright.

Challenge 2: Balancing Exercise with Other Commitments

Numerous responsibilities in life could compete for your time. Adopt a flexible attitude about working out, incorporating it easily into your everyday schedule, and making your health a top priority.

As we come to the end of our investigation into physical activity and exercise, picture a tapestry that is woven with the threads of energy, movement, and wellbeing. As you set out on this journey, embrace the transformational power of exercise and allow the rhythm of movement to become a symphony that echoes throughout your heart.

We'll explore the intricacies of food plans and nutrition in the upcoming chapter, providing your body with the sustenance it so desperately needs. Until then, may your heart's rhythm serve as a monument to the strength of movement and the human spirit's tenacity.

Stress Management Techniques

Greetings from an important stop along the way as we work to become experts at managing Congestive Heart Failure (CHF). Recognizing the significant influence of stress on our health is crucial as we traverse the complex terrain of holistic healthcare and wellbeing. Stress, which frequently lurks in the background of our everyday existence, can have a serious negative impact on both our mental and physical well-being. This is especially true in the setting of congestive heart failure (CHF), since stress can exacerbate the heart's already weakened function. But worry not, readers—in these pages, we'll explore a variety of stress-reduction strategies and mindfulness exercises that not only relieve emotional burden but also improve general wellbeing for those with CHF.

Let's clarify the current issue. Stress can have a devastating effect on our bodies and minds. It is an illusive yet constant force. The stakes are much higher when CHF is involved. Constant stress can make symptoms worse, put undue strain on the heart, and make treatment plans less successful. It's more than just feeling overburdened; there is a real risk to our well-being.

Unmanaged stress has far-reaching effects, and when combined with the complex dance of CHF, the consequences can be disastrous. Stress can set off a series of physiological reactions that can strain an already overworked heart, such as elevated blood pressure and heart rate. Moreover, it may make it more difficult for us to follow through on necessary drug schedules and lifestyle adjustments, endangering our overall health. If chronic stress is not managed, it can throw off the delicate balance of managing CHF and result in hospitalizations and exacerbations.

What then are the remedies? How do we make our way through the maze of stress and come out the other side robust and unharmed? A patchwork of mindfulness exercises and stress-reduction strategies that enable us to take back control of our emotional health holds the key to the solution. We have an extensive and diverse toolkit at our disposal, ranging from deep breathing exercises to meditation and visualisation treatments. When these routines become part of who we are, they operate as a barrier against stress's never-ending assault. They support resilience and well-being by strengthening our hearts and minds, in addition to relieving the acute load of emotional distress.

However, how can we actually implement these solutions? Acquiring knowledge of the theory is not enough; we also need to incorporate these methods into our everyday routines. Setting our mental health as a top priority is the first step toward implementation. It entails setting aside special times for self-care so that we can experience mindfulness techniques' calming embrace. It's about realising that, even in the middle of life's chaos, we are entitled to some peace and quiet.

The effectiveness of these methods is not just speculation; rather, it is supported by data and the profound firsthand accounts of innumerable people who have embraced the life-changing potential of stress-reduction approaches. Studies have demonstrated the observable advantages of mindfulness-based therapies in reducing the negative effects of stress on heart health. Moreover, the personal accounts of those who have incorporated these techniques into their daily lives serve as evidence of the significant influence they can exert. The results are enlightening and inspirational, ranging from decreased anxiety and sadness to improved general well-being.

It's important to recognise that although these methods are powerful partners in our fight against stress, they are not our only choices. It's critical to understand that every person is different and that what appeals to one may not appeal to another. Investigating non-traditional approaches, like music therapy, art therapy, or even light movement exercises, can reveal undiscovered possibilities for stress relief. The secret is to approach this healing landscape with an open mind and a sense of inquiry.

Let's not just view stress management techniques as a means of controlling one component of our wellbeing as we draw to a close our investigation of them. Rather, let us give them the respect and importance they merit, acknowledging them as essential instruments in our comprehensive strategy for managing CHF. These are not just routines; they are self-compassion and resilience rituals, seeds we plant in the rich soil of our hearts and thoughts to grow a garden of well-being.

So, dear readers, let us welcome these stress-reduction methods and mindfulness exercises with open hearts and open minds as we set off on this life-changing adventure. Let us incorporate them into our life like a tapestry, adding peaceful and serene moments to each day. Because when we do this, we not only lessen the weight of stress but also take care of the strong spirit that carries us through life's inevitable storms.

Sleep Hygiene and CHF

Greetings, reader, and welcome to the realm of holistic medicine and well-being. Here, we will explore the complex web of care for congestive heart failure (CHF), with a particular emphasis on sleep hygiene. Understanding the significance of good sleep for CHF patients is a critical component of complete care, as the intricacies of this complex illness become more apparent. So let's start this investigation and learn more about how sleep and the intricate details of CHF interact.

Think of the body as a symphony orchestra, with each member contributing in unison to produce a lovely tune of health and life. Imagine that the heart is the conductor, making sure that all the notes are played in perfect time. Even a small disturbance in the complex orchestra of CHF can throw off the entire symphony. Sleep is one such component that can upset the careful balance.

The main problem is that sleep and CHF are inversely correlated. Insomnia, restless legs syndrome, and sleep disturbances can all be brought on by congestive heart failure, and inadequate or poor-quality sleep can make the condition worse. This leads to a difficult cycle in which the illness affects sleep, which exacerbates the disease.

Imagine this loop as a violent tornado that could suck the patient into a vicious circle of exhaustion, diminished quality of life, and elevated cardiovascular event risk. If this tumultuous cycle is not treated, it can continue to deteriorate heart function and general health, which can be a strong obstacle to managing CHF effectively.

So how do we make our way through these dangerous waters? The idea of sleep hygiene, which is a group of behaviours and practises that encourage restorative and peaceful sleep, is a ray of hope. By adopting this strategy, we hope to break the cycle of disruption and open the door to better cardiac health and general wellbeing.

Setting up a regular sleep pattern is the first step towards improving sleep hygiene for people with congestive heart failure. Imagine this as the orchestra being tuned to a particular pitch, resulting in a pleasing rhythm that enables the body to anticipate and get ready for sleep. Regular sleep and wake hours are part of this regimen, which helps create a sense of predictability and calm the restless symphony of CHF.

We then explore the surroundings, the canvas on which the nighttime symphony is performed. Imagine making the most of this phase while adding a mindfulness element to make sure the bedroom is a peaceful haven. Everything from controlling temperature to reducing light and noise contributes to creating a sleep environment that is beneficial.

We come upon the idea of sensory management while navigating the nuances of good sleep hygiene. Imagine this as the soft direction of an experienced conductor leading the orchestra to a tranquil crescendo. We create a smooth transition from waking to restlessness by connecting the bed with sleep and intimacy instead of wakefulness and unrest.

We are now able to observe the transformational power of restorative sleep as these tactics are put into practise. Research has demonstrated the significant influence that optimal sleep hygiene has on the signs and prognosis of congestive heart failure (CHF), emphasising its importance as a cornerstone of all-encompassing care. Patients see a possible decrease in cardiovascular events along with decreased fatigue, elevated mood, and improved overall quality of life.

Even when we've figured out the sleep hygiene symphony, we still need to recognise that there are other options. There are several methods for treating the sleep disturbances linked to congestive heart failure (CHF), ranging from the use of positive airway pressure devices to pharmacological therapies. It is imperative, nevertheless, to address these options from a holistic standpoint and include them into a thorough framework that includes the fundamentals of good sleep hygiene.

To sum up, my dear reader, the symphony of sleep hygiene is a potent tool in the toolbox of managing chronic heart failure. Let us keep in mind that every note and every rhythm in the symphony of health and well-being is important as we continue our exploration. Accept the rhythm of healing sleep, as it is the secret to arranging a peaceful life amidst the complications of congestive heart failure.

Smoking Cessation and CHF

Greetings, reader, and welcome to this crucial point in our exploration of the intricate world of managing congestive heart failure (CHF). As we go deeper into the nuances of CHF, we need to take a moment to address a widespread problem that has a significant impact on the health of those who are facing the disease: quitting smoking.

Smoking's pervasiveness in our culture has long had a negative impact on public health. Even with everyone's knowledge of the harmful effects of smoking, smoking is still a powerful enemy, particularly for those who are suffering from CHF.

The main concern here is smoking's detrimental effects on heart health, especially when combined with congestive heart failure. Smoking is detrimental to the cardiovascular system and exacerbates the symptoms and progression of congestive heart failure (CHF), making it difficult to effectively control.

Smoking's harmful effects can cause people with CHF to suffer from a variety of serious repercussions if they are not addressed. Smoking has a staggeringly negative impact on the already weakened cardiovascular system, from hastened disease development to increased risk of life-threatening consequences.

The light of hope, quitting smoking, shines in the face of this powerful foe. People with CHF can greatly reduce the negative impact smoking has on their heart health and set themselves up for a more positive future in their fight against CHF by giving up the habit.

Adopting smoking cessation as a strategy for managing chronic heart failure necessitates a multimodal approach. It starts with a firm resolve to transform and an encouraging atmosphere that supports this decision. The arsenal of tools available to help people quit smoking is extensive and diverse, ranging from behavioural therapy and counselling to pharmaceutical assistance. Support can be customised to meet the specific needs of each user.

The effectiveness of quitting smoking in the setting of CHF is a proven fact, not just a theory. Several success stories demonstrate the life-changing potential of escaping the grip of smoking, opening a new chapter of vigour and resiliency for those with CHF.

For those with CHF, quitting smoking is the first step toward regaining heart health. However, there are other options as well, such support groups and nicotine replacement treatment, which can help along the way.

Now imagine with me the dramatic transformation that occurs when a person with CHF sets out on the life-changing journey to quit smoking. Imagine the heart, freed from the poisonous embrace of smoking, exhaling in relief as its resiliency is restored. As the smoke fades, the heart regains its strength and life, much like a delicate flower opening its petals in the first light of dawn.

Think about the complex web of behaviours and ideologies that connect smoking to a person's identity, dear reader. Liberating oneself from this complex web requires a combination of resolute determination and supportive assistance. It's not just about quitting smoking; it's about breaking free from a poisonous relationship and engaging in a meaningful act of self-care that extends well beyond the cardiovascular system.

We must pay attention to the complex dance that occurs between the mind and the body as we make our way through the maze of quitting smoking. Smoking's appeal frequently transcends physical dependence and combines with coping techniques and emotional crutches. As a result, in addition to physiological interventions, the road to smoking cessation must include psychological support and coping mechanisms that foster fortitude and resilience.

The decision to stop smoking is a critical step in the therapy of chronic heart failure (CHF), and it is evidence of the resolute resilience that drives people toward overall health. It's a proclamation of empowerment for oneself, a brave step back toward taking control of one's health and escaping the pernicious hold of smoking.

As we traverse the maze of managing chronic heart failure, dear reader, let us not undervalue the life-changing power of quitting smoking. It is a ray of hope that shows the way to a time when the heart will be free to fly without being constrained by the negative effects of smoking. With open hearts and strong resolve, let's go on this adventure because the benefits are truly life-changing.

Alcohol and CHF

Imagine yourself at a warm, well-lit restaurant, the sound of soothing conversation and soft glass clinking providing the background music. A bunch of pals get together in one corner to salute with wine on this momentous occasion. Meanwhile, a man relaxes with a refreshing beer in hand in a different area of the town after a demanding day. Our social fabric is permeated with alcohol, which is a pervasive presence during our happy, comforting, and leisurely moments.

Let me introduce you to Congestive Heart Failure (CHF), a powerful foe in the fight for ideal heart health. Millions of people are impacted by this complicated illness, which impairs the heart's capacity to pump blood effectively and sets off a chain reaction of upsetting symptoms. And then there's booze, a common indulgence that can either result in pleasant surprises or be a nice diversion. Both alcohol and CHF have unique nuances and repercussions, as they are the main characters in our storey.

The combination of alcohol and CHF presents a special dilemma. While moderate alcohol use has been associated with possible cardiovascular benefits, excessive or uncontrolled drinking can worsen the very problem that moderate alcohol use is meant to treat. So, for those negotiating the tricky terrain of CHF, where does one draw the line between indulgence and restraint?

It's critical to set strict standards that respect the fine line between pleasure and danger in order to handle this difficulty. The key to responsible alcohol drinking for those with CHF is moderation. A 12-ounce beer, a 5-ounce glass of wine, or a 1.5-ounce shot of distilled spirits is considered a single drink, according to the American Heart Association, which suggests a limit of one drink for women and two for men each day. These recommendations act as a compass, assisting patients with congestive heart failure in avoiding the dangerous waters of binge drinking.

Individuals with CHF may experience observable improvements by following these recommendations. People who practise moderation and use alcohol sparingly may be able to reduce some of the cardiovascular hazards that come with it. Additionally, by taking a balanced approach, people with CHF can feel empowered and enjoy a drink without worrying about guilt, fear, or uncertainty.

It is imperative to recognise, nonetheless, that these recommendations do not represent a universally applicable solution. It is important to consider a person's medical history, prescription history, and general health while thinking about drinking alcohol. Furthermore, cautious thought should be given to any possible interactions between alcohol and CHF drugs. In order to make well-informed decisions in this complex environment, open communication with healthcare practitioners is essential to a personalised, holistic approach.

Think about include a graphic depiction of the suggested alcohol intake limitations, such as an elegantly created infographic. This graphic tool can act as a gentle reminder, highlighting the value of moderation in an approachable and interesting way.

The relationship between alcohol and CHF captures a larger reality in healthcare: achieving well-being is a complex process with few clear-cut options. A careful dance between lifestyle decisions and medical considerations is necessary when navigating the terrain of CHF; this dance requires discernment, caution, and a hint of grace.

As we examine the complex association between alcohol and CHF in more detail, let's consider how tailored medicine and growing scientific knowledge may affect how we perceive this relationship in the future. Come along with me as we explore the complex relationship between alcohol and CHF in an effort to gain understanding, insight, and a closer understanding of the heart's workings.

Mind-Body Connection

Title: Embracing the Holistic Approaches to Congestive Heart Failure Management

As we explore the complex maze of congestive heart failure management, it is critical to acknowledge the enormous impact of the mind-body link on our general health. Imagine a calm haven where the calming embrace of relaxation techniques, the flowing yoga poses, and the soft murmurs of meditation combine to create a comprehensive healing symphony. This is the area where we integrate holistic approaches into the management of Congestive Heart Failure, driven by the steadfast conviction that true wellbeing entails the harmonic union of the mind, body, and spirit.

Set the Scene:

Imagine a serene wellness centre surrounded by the embrace of nature in this investigation of the mind-body link. Soft sunshine streams through the leaves, bathing people in need of comfort in a warm glow. Those struggling with the intricacies of congestive heart failure find solace in this place, setting out on a path that extends beyond simple medical care and includes the promotion of their mental and emotional health.

Introduce the Main Players:

Our team, a group of enthusiastic people that support the combination of holistic healthcare and wellness, is at the centre of this revolutionary approach. From physicians to health and wellness coaches to specialists in psychology, nutrition, and complementary therapies, we present a unified front committed to equipping people with the information and resources they need to thrive in the face of congestive heart failure.

Present the Challenge or Problem:

Congestive heart failure can have an emotionally and psychologically draining effect on a person, as its symptoms can also have an affect on one's physical well-being. The difficult part of treating this illness is realising that physical, emotional, and spiritual well-being all need to come together for there to be actual healing.

Detail the Approach or Solution:

In order to negotiate this complex terrain, we employ a multimodal strategy that goes beyond conventional medicine. Being able to calm the mind and promote inner peace makes meditation a vital component of our all-encompassing approach. When people combine the mild yet effective postures of yoga, they find a way to become resilient both mentally and physically. In addition, deep breathing exercises and guided imagery are examples of relaxation techniques that provide a calm haven amidst the turbulent waters of congestive heart failure.

Showcase the Results:

This integrative approach produces results that are nothing short of revolutionary. People now have a renewed sense of inner power and are able to face the difficulties presented by congestive heart failure with grace and resiliency. From a physiological perspective, we see a significant decrease in stress, which is known to aggravate the symptoms of congestive heart failure. Additionally, incorporating holistic methods improves overall quality of life by supplementing conventional medical therapies.

Analyze and Reflect:

Healing is a process that goes much beyond medical therapies when the mind-body link is incorporated into the therapy of congestive heart failure. It asks us to reflect on the unity of our being and to take care of our emotional and spiritual selves in addition to our physical selves. Although there may be objections based on doubt or the limitations of conventional medical paradigms, the observable benefits and significant changes attested to validate the effectiveness of this all-encompassing strategy.

Visual Aids (if applicable):

Imagine a tranquil setting where people find comfort in the slow, flowing poses of yoga, their motions reflecting the rhythmic dance of the natural world. Imagine the calm that surrounds them during meditation as they explore the depths of their inner self and come out on the other side feeling stronger and more at peace. The transformational effect of holistic approaches in the management of congestive heart failure is demonstrated by these graphic depictions.

Connect to the Larger Narrative or Concept:

The integration of holistic techniques fundamentally represents the harmonic convergence of mind, body, and spirit, which is the essence of comprehensive wholeness. It calls for a reconsideration of the established boundaries of healthcare and a move toward the acceptance of the whole range of human experience in the search for recovery. By acknowledging the enormous influence of the mind-body link, we open the door to a new paradigm in the treatment of congestive heart failure—one that values the complex web of life that is each of us.

Transition Thought or Question:

As we approach this life-changing experience, think about the far-reaching effects of accepting the mind-body connection in the field of medicine. How may this all-encompassing strategy spread throughout the larger field of wellness and recovery, going beyond the management of congestive heart failure? Come along with me as we set off on an enlightening journey to discover the limitless possibilities of the mind-body connection in creating a blueprint for total wellbeing.

Emotional Wellness and Support

Coping With Diagnosis

The walls feel closer than they did a few minutes ago, and the air feels thicker around you as you sit in the doctor's office. The phrase "congestive cardiac failure" carries a dark and menacing connotation. You have the impression that something has moved under your feet, and you're left juggling a flurry of feelings like shock, anxiety, and confusion. This is the point at which the course of your health journey takes an unexpected turn, my dear reader.

It's crucial to understand that being told you have congestive heart failure can be quite stressful. It's normal to experience a wide range of emotions, including shock, fear, and even sadness. It's like being caught in a storm, beaten by strong winds and pelted by rain that never stops. It is important to keep in mind that you are not alone throughout these times.

Managing the emotional and psychological effects of this diagnosis is the main challenge. The phrase "heart failure" carries a heavy burden, evoking visions of an organ that has failed and broken. Recognizing the emotional toll this can take and the potential effects on your general wellbeing is crucial.

There may be serious repercussions if these feelings are not addressed. Anxiety and stress can make your symptoms worse, which can create a vicious cycle of deteriorating health. Ignoring the emotional component of your diagnosis may make it more difficult for you to accept the required lifestyle adjustments and medical interventions, which may eventually impede your progress toward wellness.

How then can we ride out this storm and come out stronger and more resilient? The solution is to adopt useful coping mechanisms and look for the emotional support you need to stay anchored throughout this turbulent period.

Above all, give yourself permission to feel. Feeling anxious, afraid, or overwhelmed is acceptable. Feelings are a proof of your humanity, not a sign of weakness. Look for a network of support, such as family, friends, or a support group, where you can talk about your experiences and voice your worries. In addition, think about getting professional assistance from a therapist or counsellor who can support you through the emotional upheaval and teach you coping skills to get by in this unfamiliar environment.

It is impossible to overstate the importance of emotional support. Research has indicated that people with robust support networks are more adept at managing long-term medical issues, leading to enhanced general health and a higher standard of living. You are moving in the direction of holistic health by recognising and addressing the emotional effect of your diagnosis.

Finding additional resources that speak to you is crucial for adjusting to a congestive heart failure diagnosis, even though professional assistance and emotional support are also important. Joyful pursuits like music, painting, or time spent in nature can be excellent channels for letting go of pent-up feelings. In addition, mindfulness techniques like meditation and deep breathing exercises can promote inner serenity and calm the inner storm.

As you set out on this trip, keep in mind that it's not just about enduring the storm; it's also about discovering moments of beauty and solace amid the chaos. You are strong and resilient enough to handle this unfamiliar terrain, just like a robust ship crossing choppy seas.

We'll go into more detail about the all-encompassing strategy for treating congestive heart failure in the upcoming chapters, including dietary recommendations, lifestyle changes, and self-care practises. For now, though, just take a moment to recognise how strong you are to face the emotional fallout from your diagnosis. You are starting a voyage of self-awareness and resilience, and you can weather this storm and come out on the other side with renewed strength and understanding if you have the correct support system and coping mechanisms.

Family Dynamics and Relationships

Greetings, readers, and welcome to a topic that is near and dear to our hearts: the complex web of connections and family dynamics in the setting of congestive heart failure (CHF). It's critical to acknowledge the significant influence that our loved ones have on our wellbeing while we manage the difficulties of having congestive heart failure. This chapter will take us on an exploration of the intricate dance of communication, the changing responsibilities of caregivers, and the development of deep relationships within the family. The intricacies of familial relationships are crucial to our journey with CHF, just as the heart plays an important role in arranging the symphony of life within us.

The family, which is frequently referred to as the cornerstone of our support system, is a complex web of interwoven interactions, each of which adds to the resilience and strength of the entire. Within this paradigm, family members and people with CHF establish a symbiotic relationship where the ups and downs of emotions, roles, and support produce a special ecosystem of compassion and understanding.

We hope to shed light on the critical role that family dynamics and relationships play in the management and well-being of individuals with CHF by exploring the subtleties of these linkages in the context of CHF. Having a better understanding of these dynamics can help create a kind and encouraging atmosphere where patients and their loved ones can flourish in spite of the difficulties caused by CHF.

We will examine the standards of good communication, the development of caregiving responsibilities, and the development of deep relationships within the family as we go on our investigation. Our compass will be these parameters, which will lead us through the terrain of relationships and familial dynamics in the context of CHF.

Family ties are nourished by effective communication, which fosters empathy and understanding. Clear and honest communication is even more important while dealing with CHF because it creates a safe space where worries, emotions, and hopes may be expressed without shame. The family unit lives on the continual flow of communication to sustain understanding and support, just as the heart depends on blood flow to preserve life.

Similar to the complex workings of the heart, caregiving responsibilities change and adapt to meet the demands of those who have congestive heart failure. At first, caregivers might have to learn how to navigate uncharted territory while offering logistical, emotional, and physical assistance. These roles change over time as caregivers learn how to support their loved ones, console them, and find joy even in the face of hardships. The development of caring responsibilities is similar to the heart's resilience and adaptability in that it is always changing to keep things balanced in the face of difficulty.

Conversely, the difficulties brought on by CHF can also cause stress in family dynamics. Tensions within the family might arise from miscommunication, unspoken expectations, and the burden of caregiving tasks. It's important to understand that these conflicts are not specific to CHF and are frequently made worse by the challenges of managing a chronic illness. Comprehending the subtleties of these difficulties can facilitate empathetic communication and reciprocal assistance, fortifying rather than weakening family ties.

Imagine a diagram where communication lines crossover and merge to form a network of empathy and understanding inside the family. This graphic depiction highlights the significance of open and honest communication in the context of CHF by illuminating the complex webs that support family ties.

We gain significant understanding of the resiliency, flexibility, and complexity of these connections by comparing and contrasting familial dynamics and interactions. The way that relationships, communication, and caring responsibilities interact within the family is evidence of the human spirit's ability to persevere through adversity and come out on top, strengthened by a shared love and understanding.

The importance of family dynamics and relationships cannot be emphasised in the fast-paced world of today, when the demands of modern life frequently tug us in opposite directions. It is critical to acknowledge that our families' love, support, and understanding can act as an anchor during the turbulent journey of managing chronic illness as we navigate the terrain of CHF management. Family ties have always been important and continue to be a source of strength and optimism in a time when technology has the power to unite and divide us.

We'll discuss resilience and self-care in the context of CHF in the upcoming subchapter, and we'll look at how people and their families can develop inner strength and wellbeing in the face of chronic illness. Until then, keep in mind that the soul is sustained by the harmonic dance of familial ties, which fosters love and fortitude in the face of hardship, much as the heart needs a regular rhythm to survive.

With love and compassion,

Dr. Ankita Kashyap

Peer Support and Community

One of the most important things we learn as we go through the Congestive Heart Failure Mastery Bible's pages is the value of community and support in helping us deal with the challenges of managing congestive heart failure. Imagine this: a colourful tapestry of people, each with their own difficulties and tales to tell, bound together by a shared resilience and optimism. For CHF patients, peer support and community are fundamentally this: a lifeline of comprehension, empathy, and common experiences.

Let's enter the calm environment of a support group gathering, where there is a strong sense of unity in the air. People from many walks of life come together here, united by the common experience of managing congestive heart failure. A haven of understanding and connection, the room hums with knowing glances and murmured discussions.

The patients themselves, each with their own medical background, struggles, and victories, are among the main characters. One such woman is Sarah, a vibrant 50-year-old who, following her diagnosis, found comfort in her relationships with other CHF warriors. Then there is Michael, a loving father and husband who learned the invaluable importance of peer support in managing the psychological effects of his illness. Not to be overlooked are the unsung heroes who contribute their knowledge and steadfast support to the community: the nurses, caregivers, and other medical professionals.

The main obstacle is the emotional strain and sense of loneliness that frequently follow a diagnosis of CHF. Anxiety, doubt, and overwhelm are powerful emotions that can cast a shadow over achieving holistic wellbeing. Patients confront a variety of challenges in managing their congestive heart failure (CHF), including the need for unshakable dedication to lifestyle adjustments, medication adherence, and mental well-being.

The community's mutual support and shared experiences have a great impact, which leads to the solution. People can access a vital source of empathy and motivation via peer mentorship programmes, internet forums, and support groups. These forums provide a secure setting for discussing worries, successes, and useful advice for overcoming the challenges of daily life with CHF. Additionally, patients are given a comprehensive toolkit for managing their disease through the integration of holistic healthcare and wellness coaching, which promotes a sense of empowerment and self-efficacy.

Peer support and community involvement have positively transformational effects. Patients report a noticeable reduction in their anxiety and feelings of loneliness that has been replaced with a renewed sense of resilience and belonging. According to studies, people who actively participate in peer support programmes had better mental health, better medication adherence, and a stronger sense of agency over their disease management. Families and caregivers are also affected by the ripple effect, as they gain from the community's resources and support.

As we consider these case studies, we get important insights into the restorative potential of interpersonal relationships. The mutual support among members of the group not only mitigates the psychological effects of CHF but also cultivates a feeling of solidarity and resolve. While some may express worries about the possibility of false information in peer support groups, when professional supervision and evidence-based procedures are followed, the advantages of emotional support and shared experiences greatly exceed the risks.

Imagine graphs showing how peer support improves a patient's quality of life, adherence to medication, and mental health. These graphic depictions reaffirm the observable advantages of community involvement, reafirming its position as a fundamental component of comprehensive CHF care.

The storey of community and peer support strikes a deep chord with the main idea of holistic treatment and wellness. It emphasises how closely mental health, social support, and physical health are intertwined and highlights how important it is to address CHF holistically. Each component harmonises to provide a melody of resiliency and hope, much like in a symphony.

Let's consider this as we wrap out our investigation of peer support and community: in a society that frequently feels fractured and alienating, what better gift can we give than the steadfast understanding and support of a group that helps us get through our lowest points?

Peer support and community are colourful threads that weave together stories of bravery, resiliency, and common humanity in the fabric of CHF management. The real skill of managing congestive heart failure is revealed in these relationships; it does not happen in isolation but rather with the support of a group of people who are living examples of the resilience of the human spirit.

Therapeutic Outlets

It is impossible to overstate the significant influence that mental health has on general health in the intricate and frequently daunting field of congestive heart failure management. Since the human heart is a powerful organ in both the physical and emotional domains, managing it requires a comprehensive strategy that recognises the connection between the mind, body, and spirit.

Imagine a busy hospital ward where congestive heart failure patients are juggling a variety of psychological and physical difficulties. There's a tangible sense of unease and fear in the air as these people struggle with the difficult nature of their illness. It is in this environment that we demonstrate the efficacy of therapeutic outlets, providing a ray of hope and recovery in the midst of the storm.

Our approach to managing congestive heart failure is based on the knowledge that our patients are active contributors to their own health rather than passive beneficiaries of medical care. In my capacity as this ship's captain, I lead a committed group of professionals who each bring a specialisation to the table. Our team comprises professionals that specialise in nutrition, psychology, creative therapy, and wellness coaching. Our goal is to offer a holistic support system that surpasses conventional medical interventions.

One cannot emphasise the psychological toll that congestive heart failure takes. As they come to terms with the reality of their illness, many patients struggle with anxiety, depression, and a sense of loss. Furthermore, physical symptoms brought on by stress and mental strain might worsen, resulting in a vicious cycle that compromises general health. It became clear in the face of these obstacles that the complex demands of our patients could not be adequately met by regular medical procedures alone.

Let me introduce you to therapeutic outlets: a myriad of artistic and expressive mediums that are a spiritual healer. For example, art therapy offers a secure environment in which patients can express their innermost thoughts and feelings without being limited by language. On the other side, music therapy uses melody and rhythm's healing properties to provide comfort and an outlet for emotions. Through journaling, creative writing, and other self-expression exercises, patients can engage in introspection and learn to face and negotiate their emotional landscapes.

In order to help patients achieve inner calm and ground themselves in the present, our method also includes breathing exercises, guided imagery, and mindfulness techniques. These techniques are essential parts of our all-encompassing approach to empowering patients on their path to holistic wellbeing, not just extras to conventional medical care.

Our patients' experiences with therapeutic outlets have been nothing short of miraculous. In one particularly moving instance, an art therapy patient who had long battled anxiety discovered comfort and renewed resilience. Her ability to externalise her anxieties and concerns through painting turned into a kind of catharsis that eventually improved her general emotional well-being. A man who had struggled with depression also found solace in music therapy, finding that even the act of plucking a guitar could provide him with emotional release and relief.

Beyond isolated incidents, we have seen a general change in our patients' emotional terrain. Our community has experienced a blossoming of friendship and mutual support as patients participate in group creative sessions and exchange personal narratives. A more robust and capable patient population has been made possible by the reduction of the emotional weight that earlier weighed heavily.

Although there is no denying the benefits of therapeutic outlets, it is important to recognise that they are not a cure-all. They are a component of a wider healthcare system, not a replacement for conventional medical treatments. Furthermore, integrating various sources calls for a personalised and nuanced approach, acknowledging that what works for one patient might not work for another.

Envision a painting filled with vivid colours, where every brushstroke conveys a tale of tenacity and optimism. Imagine a circle of patients with their voices blending into a therapeutic symphony and their hands plucking guitars. Words cannot adequately convey the value of therapeutic outlets, but these images do.

Fundamentally, the inclusion of therapeutic outlets reflects our approach's larger philosophy that healing is a comprehensive process that takes into account all aspects of the human experience. We respect our patients' innate humanity by acknowledging the emotional aspects of congestive heart failure and the fact that their wellbeing goes well beyond the pages of medical records and diagnostic testing.

As we venture into the unexplored realm of managing congestive heart failure, let us consider: what other innovative and healing paths could be guiding lights for our patients? Furthermore, how can we keep incorporating emotional health into the core of medical care?

The path to healing is complex, and we may genuinely encourage our patients to flourish in the midst of hardship by integrating physical, emotional, and spiritual approaches in a harmonic manner. We shall explore the complex dance of holistic healing in greater detail in the upcoming chapters, telling a storey that highlights the human spirit's resiliency.

Seeking Professional Help

We frequently concentrate on the physical aspects of Congestive Heart Failure (CHF) management, which includes nutrition, exercise, and medications. These are all vital parts of the great symphony of CHF management. However, what about the psychological and emotional toll that chronic illness takes? The silent partners that frequently go unappreciated are the feelings of anxiety, dread, and uncertainty. At this point, professional counselling and therapy play a crucial role in providing a lighthouse through the emotional maze that comes with having CHF.

Now let's get to the core of the issue. Living with CHF involves mental and emotional struggles in addition to physical ones. One's emotional health may suffer greatly from the ongoing observation, the lifestyle changes, and the anxiety of flare-ups. These mental responsibilities might weigh as much, if not more, than the physical pains.

These mental baggage have the power to cloud every part of life if they are not handled. An ongoing state of worry and anxiety may permeate every aspect of your life, impacting your relationships, your productivity at work, and your general well-being. This is the quiet cost of having CHF, a cost that cannot be entirely mitigated by medicine or physical therapy.

Nevertheless, readers need not worry, for competent counselling and therapy is a bright light amidst this confusing and frequently turbulent world. Think of these experts as the sherpa helping you navigate the dangerous highs and lows of your emotional turmoil and offering a steady hand to get you out of the maze and into the light.

Getting professional assistance is a brave step toward taking back control of your emotional health, not a sign of weakness. It's like calling in a group of expert weavers to repair the ragged mental tapestry and weave in the strands of optimism, resiliency, and hope.

What then does getting expert assistance involve? It involves more than just opening up to a sympathetic listener while seated in a comfortable office. It's about arming yourself with the knowledge and techniques necessary to successfully negotiate the emotional terrain of CHF. A range of techniques are included in professional counselling and therapy, such as mindfulness-based interventions, cognitive behavioural therapy, and supportive counselling catered to your individual requirements.

You and your mental health practitioner must work together to put these therapy techniques into practise. Together, you will investigate the root causes of your emotional discomfort, create coping strategies for anxiety and depression, and build a resilient mentality that will enable you to meet the difficulties of CHF head-on.

"But how can I know if professional counselling and therapy will genuinely make a difference?" is probably what's on your mind right now. Permit me to discuss the significant effects that these actions may have with you. Studies indicate that participation in professional counselling and therapy significantly lowers anxiety and sadness in patients with congestive heart failure (CHF), improves adherence to treatment plans, and improves overall quality of life.

These therapies can also be a crucial adjunct to the physical components of managing congestive heart failure (CHF), resulting in a holistic strategy that supports the body and the mind. It's similar to taking care of a fragile garden; without nourishing the soil below the flowers, you can't expect them to flourish. In a same spirit, taking care of your mental health is the soil in which resilience and strength grow.

Of course, there are other options besides professional counselling and therapy for dealing with emotional distress related to congestive heart failure. Other strategies, such self-help methods, relaxation techniques, and support groups, can be excellent providers of emotional support. These options can support professional interventions by adding more emotional support layers to strengthen your wellbeing.

Ultimately, getting expert assistance for the emotional discomfort, anxiety, and depression brought on by CHF is an essential part of your all-encompassing care plan for the condition, not just a choice. It's the brave act of reaching out to help lift the burden of emotional distress, enabling you to move through the CHF terrain with hope and resilience.

So, my readers, keep in mind that professional counselling and therapy are faithful allies that provide comfort, support, and guidance through the emotional ups and downs as we continue our journey through the maze of CHF treatment. Accept these allies, and with unflinching strength and optimism, we will traverse the emotional terrain of CHF together.

Spirituality and Faith

There are strands in the complex tapestry of life that connect us to something that is not of this world, outside the domain of science and medicine. These threads are the components of faith and spirituality, which have the capacity to comfort the soul and lift it above hardship. When we explore the world of Congestive Heart Failure (CHF), it is clear that there is more to this complicated illness than meets the eye. We can start to understand the significant impact of spirituality and faith in the treatment of CHF by taking a holistic approach that takes into account the mind, body, and spirit.

Picture a calm hospital room with ambient lighting that is soothing and the sound of medical equipment hums softly in the background. Here, we meet Ms. Evelyn, a 65-year-old lady with a history of congestive heart failure. Her thoughts appear to be whisked away by the soft breeze that blows through the open window as she sits beside it and looks out at the world outside. She exudes serenity and inner strength in spite of the difficulties she encounters; her resilience is fostered by her unshakable spirituality and faith.

For a number of years, retired school teacher Ms. Evelyn has been navigating CHF. Along with periods of anxiety and uncertainty, her path has also been characterised by steadfast faith and a strong bond with her spiritual beliefs. Beside Ms. Evelyn is her medical staff, a committed set of experts who understand the crucial role that spirituality and faith play in her comprehensive care. They present a united front by combining their deep understanding of the human spirit with their medical skills.

In addition to managing her physical symptoms, Ms. Evelyn's path with CHF has involved navigating the emotional and spiritual upheaval that frequently accompanies chronic illness. People with CHF may have significant life challenges due to the weight of uncertainty, fear of the unknown, and existential dilemmas raised by mortality.

Ms. Evelyn's healthcare team has integrated spirituality and faith into her care plan, acknowledging the complex nature of the situation. They have encouraged Ms. Evelyn to rely on her faith for strength, turn to prayer for comfort, and partake in activities that align with her spiritual values through frank and kind discussions. They have also included mindfulness and meditation practises that complement her religious beliefs, which promote calmness and inner serenity.

Incorporating spirituality and faith into Ms. Evelyn's treatment plan has had a significant impact. She talks of having a newfound sense of purpose and inner fortitude that have given her the strength to overcome the difficulties brought on by CHF. She no longer feels as anxious and has a calmness that surpasses the limitations of her illness. Her physical problems have also improved, which is evidence of the connection between the mind, body, and spirit.

Thinking back on Ms. Evelyn's journey serves as a reminder of the significant impact that spirituality and religion have on the medical field. The human spirit is resilient, as seen by the ways in which spiritual beliefs can offer consolation, purpose, and strength in the face of disease. But it's important to understand that spirituality is very personal, and integrating religion into care planning ought to be done so with consideration and respect for each person's unique views.

Visual aids in this section could include peaceful pictures that inspire a feeling of spirituality and faith, like a peaceful natural environment, a meditation area lighted by candles, or a person practising a spiritual activity that is in line with their beliefs.

The incorporation of spirituality and religion into CHF care is a microcosm of the larger movement in healthcare toward a more holistic approach. In light of the fact that true healing encompasses the entirety of the human experience, it emphasises the significance of treating the emotional and spiritual elements of illness in addition to its physical manifestations.

Let's consider the importance of spirituality and faith in the context of healthcare as we go through the pages of "The Congestive Heart Failure Mastery Bible: Your Blueprint for Complete Congestive Heart Failure Management.' Since chronic illness has a significant impact on a person's general health and well-being, how can we continue to support their spiritual well-being? Come along with me as we investigate these issues and learn more about the transforming potential of holistic treatment.

Resilience and Hope

As we go out on this trip over the complex terrain of managing congestive heart failure, it is critical to accept the hope and resilience that can be developed in the face of this difficult illness. We find inspiration that goes beyond the clinical setting and serves as a lighthouse for people navigating the challenges of congestive heart failure in the tales of victory, tenacity, and the unbreakable human spirit.

Imagine yourself in a calm hospital room that is illuminated by the gentle morning light. A patient lies in a corner with their loved ones and a committed medical staff around them. This serves as the background against which the human soul, despite congestive heart disease, demonstrates its amazing capacity for resiliency and hope.

Despite being diagnosed with congestive heart failure, Sarah is a lively and enthusiastic person who exudes a contagious enthusiasm for life. Her medical team, which consists of nurses, holistic wellness specialists, and cardiologists, creates a network of support aimed at enabling her to take charge of her path. Together, they create a treatment plan that includes holistic approaches to fostering hope and resilience in addition to medical measures.

The main obstacles in Sarah's case are not just managing her congestive heart failure but also maintaining her quality of life and fostering her mental and emotional health. Significant restrictions are imposed by congestive heart disease, and even the most optimistic people might become depressed due to fear of the unknown.

The strategy used to address this difficulty was holistic treatment, which included dietary and lifestyle adjustments, individual diet planning, psychological counselling, and a wide range of self-care and coping mechanisms. Sarah was gently led down a path that nourished her optimism and honoured her resiliency, enabling her to take an active role in her own care process.

Integrating holistic wellness techniques, such as gentle yoga, focused meditation, and the investigation of substitutes for self-care, were cornerstones of her path. These enhanced conventional medical procedures, resulting in a comprehensive strategy that honoured her as a person, not just a patient.

This strategy produced nothing short of extraordinary results. Sarah found a source of inner resilience in addition to gaining a better comprehension of her illness. She revelled in the small pleasures of life, comforted by the warmth of her loved ones and her body, mind, and soul-nurturing practises.

Her medical team saw measurable improvements in her general health, backed by statistics, illustrating the transformative potential of holistic care in the context of managing congestive heart failure. Sarah's narrative served as a ray of hope for others, demonstrating that perseverance can thrive under the most trying conditions.

Sarah's path provides significant understanding of the human spirit's resiliency. It makes us think about the ability of holistic care to foster optimism and fortitude in the face of congestive heart failure as well as in all facets of healthcare. It emphasises how crucial it is to adopt a holistic strategy that values the unique person and acknowledges the connection between the mind, body, and spirit.

Sarah's tale serves as a powerful reminder that hope is an active force that can be developed rather than a passive bystander as we traverse the challenges of managing congestive heart disease. It pushes us to investigate novel strategies that uphold the human spirit's capacity for resiliency and inspire hope in the hearts of persons dealing with health issues.

Envision a graph that shows both the clinical indicators of improvement and the non-quantifiable dimensions of wellbeing; this would serve as a visual depiction of the transforming potential of holistic treatment when it comes to managing congestive heart failure.

Sarah's journey is a perfect example of how the individual tales of everyone of us are the beating hearts of the larger storey of healthcare. It emphasises how important it is to provide comprehensive care, celebrate resilience, and foster hope as a necessary part of the healing process.

As we delve deeper into the complex world of managing congestive heart failure, let's consider this: How can we help people who are struggling with their health feel resilient and hopeful, creating a care system that honours the fullness of the human spirit? Come along as we explore the human spirit's resiliency and the transforming potential of holistic healing.

Supportive Care and Practical Strategies

Care Coordination and Advocacy

Greetings, readers! Now let's get down to business: care coordination and advocacy play a critical part in the all-encompassing management of congestive heart failure (CHF). It's critical to comprehend the significant effects of navigating the healthcare system, getting access to resources, and fighting for comprehensive care for our patients as we set out on this path toward complete CHF management. We will examine the complex network of care coordination and advocacy in this subchapter, as well as the issues, repercussions, and—above all—solutions that have the potential to revolutionise the field of CHF management.

First, let's establish the scene. Patients with CHF frequently experience a plethora of complications in the maze-like world of contemporary healthcare, ranging from disjointed care paths to the bewildering number of options. It can be likened to setting out on a trek through a dense forest, where every turn brings a new obstacle, navigating this complex web. The main problem is that patients are exposed to inadequate care and fragmented support networks due to a lack of efficient coordination and lobbying.

The implications of this disjointed approach are extensive, and they may have an effect on the core of a patient's health. Patients may have fragmented management plans, a sense of isolation along their journey, and delayed access to necessary treatments in the absence of efficient care coordination and advocacy. Their emotional and psychological fortitude are also negatively impacted, which has a knock-on effect on their physical health and affects every part of their existence.

Let's now shed light on the future course and potential fixes to close the gaps and establish a strong support network for CHF sufferers. The foundation of this approach is the idea of holistic care coordination and advocacy, in which the patient is positioned at the centre of a multidisciplinary team and all members collaborate to provide a harmonious level of care. This method incorporates a thorough plan that transcends medical procedures and embraces the philosophy of wellness and holistic healthcare.

This approach is implemented like a delicate dance, with each move being intentional and meaningful. It starts with the formation of a cooperative care team made up of physicians, specialists in health and wellbeing, and patient advocates. With the help of a multidisciplinary team, every aspect of the patient's journey—from nutritional planning and lifestyle adjustments to psychological support and coping mechanisms—is carefully attended to. We provide a safety net that supports the full person, not just the ailment, by tying together a web of care that goes beyond the boundaries of conventional medicine.

As we follow this road, we must highlight the transformative results that this strategy may produce. Through the adoption of comprehensive care coordination and advocacy, we observe our patients' transformation from a state of vulnerability to one of empowerment. With the information and assistance they need to successfully negotiate the healthcare system, patients take an active role in their treatment. This empowerment affects not just their physical health but also their emotional and psychological well-being, having a knock-on impact that affects all aspect of their lives.

Even while this strategy provides a ray of optimism, it's critical to recognise that there are other options. Every path has advantages of its own, and we can only truly comprehend the terrain ahead of us if we thoroughly investigate these options. But the comprehensive approach to advocacy and care coordination speaks to the core of our values, which are to support our patients' overall well-being and accept their journey with empathy and understanding.

Every thread in the care coordination and advocacy tapestry has a purpose and comes together to form a support network that goes beyond the confines of conventional healthcare. While navigating this complex network, let's consider the significant effects of our actions:

the ability of holistic care to transform and the resilience it instils in our patients' hearts.

My dear readers, let us embrace Maya Angelou's great wisdom as we go out on this journey of care coordination and advocacy: "People will forget what you did, they will forget what you said, but they will never forget how you made them feel." Let's forge a route that addresses physical ailments while also fostering spiritual well-being, leaving a compassionate and empowering legacy in the field of CHF care.

Financial Resources and Assistance

Welcome to the subject of financial resources and support accessible to patients to help with their healthcare needs. This is a topic that is sometimes disregarded but has great importance in the management of congestive heart failure (CHF). As we begin this investigation, it is critical to recognise the complex obstacles that CHF patients must overcome, both in terms of their overall health and the financial strain associated with treating this illness.

The main problem at hand is the significant financial burden that CHF patients and their families bear. The expense of medical treatment, prescription drugs, and continuing care can quickly mount, leading to a great deal of worry and concern. Trying to keep afloat as the waves of bills loom large is like sailing through a storm.

Let's now explore the effects of this financial hardship. The weight of medical expenses can force people to make tough decisions and compromises if it is not addressed. Patients may have to forgo necessary medical care or prescription drugs, endangering their health and general wellbeing. It's similar to a fine balance that may have significant effects on the way CHF is managed overall if it were to be upset.

But do not worry; help is on the way. In order to relieve the burden of healthcare costs and guarantee access to essential medical treatment and drugs, a plethora of financial resources and assistance programmes are available to CHF patients. These initiatives provide a lifeline to individuals in need and act as rays of hope in the frequently muddy waters of healthcare expenditures.

The process of putting these answers into practise entails figuring out which resources and help programmes are accessible. To find and use these priceless resources, proactive collaboration with social workers, financial counsellors, and healthcare professionals is necessary. Finding the hidden jewels that can ease financial burdens and open the door to efficient CHF management is like to going on a treasure hunt.

It's encouraging to see the excellent results that have been seen when evaluating the efficacy of these financial resources and aid initiatives. By using these services, patients have reported a major decrease in financial stress, which has allowed them to concentrate on their health and wellbeing. It seems like a burden being lifted off their shoulders, enabling them to go through their CHF journey more confidently and easily.

Even while these programmes provide a lot of help, it's crucial to recognise that there are other options. Some patients might find it helpful to look into other financial support options, such as pharmaceutical assistance programmes, charity foundations, or patient advocacy groups. People can further strengthen their network of financial assistance by customising their strategy to fit their unique requirements and circumstances by taking these choices into consideration.

In conclusion, in the frequently turbulent world of healthcare prices, the availability of financial resources and aid for CHF sufferers is a ray of hope. By utilising these tools, people can lessen their financial burden and guarantee that they have access to necessary prescription drugs and medical care. It serves as a lifeline for people facing the challenges of managing chronic heart failure and is evidence of the strength of support and unity.

Remember that you are not alone as we continue to read through "The Congestive Heart Failure Mastery Bible: Your Blueprint for Complete Congestive Heart Failure Management." Resources, help, and a supportive community are ready to help you navigate this difficult terrain. By working together, we can successfully manage the financial aspects of CHF, enabling people to put their health and wellbeing first without having to worry about money.

Home Care and Assistance

For those managing the challenges of congestive heart failure, home is truly where the heart is. Establishing a secure and supportive environment inside our homes is essential as we navigate the complexities of treating this condition. The practical methods and tools for providing home care and support, maximising comfort and safety in the home, and eventually promoting a sense of well-being for those with congestive heart failure are covered in this subchapter.

Our main goal is to provide you with the knowledge and resources you need to turn your house into a haven that aids in your management of congestive heart failure. By putting these tactics into practise, you'll create a setting that supports your general wellbeing and gives you the empowerment you need.

This method's simplicity is what makes it so beautiful. There are no long lists of supplies or requirements; all that is needed is a readiness to adapt and a desire to create a cosy and healing environment.

Let's begin with a quick rundown of the stages in this process of transformation. We'll look at your home's physical features, from making it more peaceful and orderly to making it safer. We'll also explore the psychological and emotional aspects, comprehending how your surroundings affect your mental and emotional health.

Let's start by concentrating on the physical surroundings. Promoting serenity and lowering stress levels require a calm, well-organized environment. Decluttering your living room, adding natural features like plants or light, and creating spaces set apart for rest and relaxation are all worthwhile ideas. These small but powerful adjustments can have a big impact on your general wellbeing.

Turning now to the safety component, you should make sure that all possible risks are identified in your property. This could entail making sure walkways are clear and easy to navigate, putting in handrails, and tying down area rugs. You should also think about putting in place a system for keeping necessary medical supplies close at hand and arranging prescriptions. By taking these precautions, you can feel safer and have peace of mind knowing that your house is a safe and encouraging place.

Let's now examine the psychological and emotional aspects of home help and care. Your house ought to be a sanctuary where you can find peace and comfort from the difficulties of living with congestive heart failure. Think about adding features that make you happy and comfortable, such making a comfortable reading corner, putting treasured memories on display, or surrounding yourself with inspirational art. These thoughtful gestures can have a significant effect on your mental health by fostering optimism and resiliency.

It's crucial that you approach this life-changing experience with an open mind and an adaptable mindset as you set out on it. Your home should be a reflection of your unique personality and goals, so pay attention to the particular demands and preferences that speak to you individually. Seeking the advice of loved ones and medical professionals is crucial when implementing these adjustments, as their viewpoints and support can be invaluable.

Examining or Verifying: How are you going to determine whether your efforts were successful? It will practically be felt in the air. Your house will exude peace and quiet, and you'll discover that it not only enhances your physical health but also feeds your soul. You'll be able to observe how these adjustments have affected your day-to-day activities as you go around your house feeling more at ease and comfortable.

In the event that difficulties arise, keep in mind that this is a dynamic process. Seize the chance to review and improve your strategy, drawing ideas from a range of sources and people who can provide direction and encouragement. You are on an ongoing investigation to create a caring home environment, and with each step you take, you go closer to having a place that genuinely epitomises safety, comfort, and well-being.

Remember that you have the ability to create a haven in your house that will help you during your journey with congestive heart failure as we negotiate the challenges of home care and assistance. By adding aspects of peace, security, and emotional support to your house, you are not only making it a place where you can retreat to, but also a place that will strengthen your will to survive. Your house becomes a symbol of your steadfast character and your dedication to overall wellbeing.

We will continue to delve into the many facets of managing Congestive Heart Failure in the pages that follow, providing you with insights and techniques to help you along the way. Together, we will discover the recipe for managing congestive heart failure completely while embracing a wholistic mindset that nourishes your body, mind, and soul.

Transportation and Mobility

Greetings, my dear reader. It is important to acknowledge the complexity of congestive heart failure as we begin our journey together through the complexities of managing this condition. We've talked about how critical physical activity is, how important mental health is, and how important diet is. Now, let's talk about mobility and transportation, a subject that exudes independence and freedom.

Everyday existence is a dance between dreams and destinations, a symphony of motion. But this dance can turn into a scary waltz for anyone navigating the maze of congestive heart failure. For CHF patients, mobility and transportation issues are as different as the patients themselves. Every step, whether it's climbing stairs or using public transportation, might seem like a mountain to climb.

The main problem is the restrictions on physical stamina that CHF imposes. Easy chores that you used to take for granted can become difficult, and your freedom of movement may seem like a thing of the past. People may become confined to their houses due to a fear of exhaustion or dyspnea, which can lower their quality of life and make them feel alone.

There may be serious repercussions if the mobility and transportation issue is not resolved. Patients with CHF may experience social isolation, despair, and a sense of powerlessness that overpowers their lively spirits. Their everyday experiences may be negatively impacted by the loss of freedom, which can have an effect on both their mental and physical health.

Do not be alarmed; there is hope for the future. Mobility aids, accessible transportation options, and tools for preserving independence can act as rays of hope, shedding light on the way to restored autonomy and self-assurance.

Let's start by discussing accessible transportation. For CHF patients, community transport programmes, customised van services, and paratransit services can be a lifeline, enabling them to get where they're going in comfort and easily. Furthermore, the employment of mobility assistance devices, such wheelchairs, walkers, or canes, can provide immeasurable assistance, allowing people to move around with more confidence.

Moreover, including lifestyle adjustments might also be crucial to improving mobility. Gentle physical activities, like yoga or tai chi, can improve balance and strength while lessening the physical strain of regular tasks. Improved energy levels can also be a result of adopting a heart-healthy diet and controlling fluid intake, which can provide a strong basis for an active lifestyle.

The lives of CHF patients have undergone incredible changes as a result of the application of these remedies. People who have adopted accessible transportation alternatives and made use of mobility aids have felt a renewed feeling of freedom and autonomy. They've discovered a newfound love for life and are going on trips and experiences that they previously thought were unachievable. Many have experienced an increase in their physical resilience by incorporating lifestyle improvements, which enables them to navigate their environment with revitalised energy and vitality.

Even if these methods have shown to be revolutionary, it's crucial to acknowledge that there are other options. Support groups provide a supportive environment where people can share their stories and learn from others who have experienced similar things. Some people can find solace in the help of in-home caregivers, who can offer customised aid to ease everyday tasks.

Mobility and freedom are the threads that connect a sense of purpose and belonging in the fabric of life. CHF patients can overcome seemingly insurmountable limits by adopting accessible transportation options, incorporating mobility aids, and cultivating a resilient lifestyle. As we proceed, let us not forget that the movement symphony never stops, beckoning us to dance with fresh strength and grace.

Nutritional Support and Meal Planning

Welcome to the realm of integrative medicine and wellness, where managing congestive heart failure is mostly dependent on diet and nutrition (CHF). We will examine the critical role that meal planning and nutritional support play in the lives of CHF patients in this subchapter, providing a thorough manual to guarantee that they have access to wholesome meals and dietary support for optimum health. Let us keep in mind that food is more than just physical nourishment for our bodies as we set out on this journey—it is essential to our total health, healing, and rejuvenation.

Establish the Goal:

Our goal is very clear: to provide CHF patients with the information and tools they need to make wise food decisions that promote overall vitality and heart health. By the time you finish this chapter, you will know how to make heart-healthy, well-balanced meal plans and how to get individualised nutritional assistance services.

List the Necessary Materials or Prerequisites:

All you need to start this journey is the will to put your health first, an open mind, and a willingness to adopt new eating habits. A solid foundation for this investigation will also come from having a fundamental understanding of macronutrients and their significance in heart health.

Begin with a Broad Overview:

Let us first recognise the importance of this undertaking before getting into the specifics of meal planning and nutritional support. Nutrition is essential for reducing fluid retention, promoting general well-being, and maximising heart function in the context of CHF management. Through the development of a comprehensive meal plan and the utilisation of targeted nutritional assistance, we can improve the quality of life for individuals with congestive heart failure and create opportunities for a healthy, heart-healthy future.

Dive into Detailed Steps:

Recognizing the Dietary Needs of Patients with CHF

To create a heart-healthy meal plan, one must first ascertain the dietary needs of individuals with chronic heart failure (CHF). This entails a sophisticated comprehension of sodium consumption, fluid restriction, and the deliberate balancing of macronutrients to bolster cardiac performance while avoiding excessive stress on the cardiovascular system.

Creating a Balanced Meal Plan

Having a strong understanding of the nutrients needed, the next step is to design a meal plan that is balanced and compliant with the CHF patient's dietary restrictions. A heart-healthy diet's main components are a variety of nutrient-dense foods with a focus on fruits, vegetables, whole grains, lean meats, and healthy fats. Furthermore, mindful eating techniques and portion control are essential for promoting general wellbeing.

Accessing Nutritional Support Services

Patients with CHF can benefit greatly from nutritional support programmes, which give them access to qualified dietitians, nutritional counselling, and specialised meal planning tools. By using these services, people can get individualised advice based on their particular dietary requirements, ensuring that they get the help they need to succeed on their heart-healthy journey.

Offer Tips and Warnings:

It's crucial to approach dietary changes with patience and an open mind as you go out on the journey of meal planning and nutritional support. Try out new recipes, enjoy the wide variety of flavours that whole foods have to offer, and look for local resources that can offer more encouragement and inspiration. Additionally, while choosing packaged or processed foods, exercise caution and keep an eye out for hidden sources of sodium. Recall that when it comes to nutrition and heart health, little adjustments can have a big impact.

Testing or Validation:

The formulation of a customised, heart-healthy meal plan that satisfies the unique nutritional requirements of CHF patients serves as validation for the successful completion of this step. Furthermore, reaching out for nutritional support services and having the confidence to make educated food decisions are concrete indicators of advancement on this life-changing path.

Troubleshooting (optional):

If obstacles arise during the process, such as managing dietary limitations or feeling overburdened by the thought of organising meals, keep in mind that you are not by yourself. Seek assistance from medical professionals, neighbourhood associations, and other individuals with CHF who may provide direction and motivation. You'll find it helpful to embrace a resilient and adaptable mindset as you work through the complexities of meal planning and nutritional support.

Let us consider the significant role that nutrition plays in managing CHF as we wrap up this subchapter. In the same way that a gardener provides intentional and thoughtful care to the soil in order to generate a rich harvest, we too need to nourish our bodies. We may build a foundation of vitality, resilience, and heart-healthy living by embracing the power of nutrition and utilising the resources that support our dietary journey. Let us keep in mind that every meal is an opportunity to nourish not only the body but also the soul, paving the way for a life replete with health and vitality, as we continue our research of holistic healthcare and wellbeing.

Legal and Ethical Considerations

Title: Managing Congestive Heart Failure While Managing the Law and Ethics

It is essential to traverse the very complex and even intimidating realm of legal and ethical issues as we set out on this quest to master the management of congestive heart failure (CHF). We will simplify the issues of healthcare decision-making, advance directives, and patient rights in this chapter, providing insight into how to provide comprehensive and compassionate care for people with CHF.

Let's set the scene before we get into the legal and ethical nuances. In the context of managing congestive heart failure, the healthcare landscape encompasses more than only medical intervention. Empathy, respect for patient autonomy, and the careful balancing act between patient rights and therapeutic imperatives are all interwoven into this tapestry.

The main concern here is the need to make sure that medical procedures adhere to the moral precepts of beneficence, non-maleficence, autonomy, and fairness. When dealing with a chronic and progressive illness like congestive heart failure (CHF), how can we make sure that our patients receive the best care possible while yet honouring their autonomy and preferences?

There will be serious repercussions if we ignore these moral questions. When these important factors are neglected, it can lead to patient discontent, weakened confidence in the healthcare system, and moral conundrums for medical professionals. Moreover, failing to recognise the autonomy and rights of patients can make those in charge of CHF feel powerless.

Our suggested strategy for overcoming these obstacles is based on a patient-centric methodology that combines advance care planning, transparent communication, and a thorough comprehension of ethical concepts. We may create a road toward thorough and compassionate

CHF care by giving patients the information they need to make decisions and honouring their autonomy.

Talking openly and honestly with patients about their beliefs, treatment choices, and advance directives is the first step towards putting this approach into practise. As a result, a collaborative approach to care can be implemented, guaranteeing that the patient's voice will always be central to the decision-making process. Creating a supportive atmosphere that recognises the psychological and emotional aspects of managing CHF is also essential to this process.

Research indicates that patients who participate in prior care planning enjoy a higher quality of life, less anxiety, and a feeling of control over their medical path. We can establish a helpful ecosystem that supports the overall well-being of people managing CHF in addition to addressing the medical elements of the condition by including these ethical issues into CHF management.

While there are several models for ethical decision-making and advance care planning in the medical field, ours places a strong emphasis on a customised and patient-driven approach. Standardized care directives or a more directed approach to decision-making are examples of other alternatives, although they could not adequately represent the complex requirements and preferences of people with CHF.

It's like navigating through unknown waters as we make our way through the ethical and legal environment of CHF management. The destination—a healthcare system that respects patient autonomy and promotes compassionate care—beckons us even though the path is full with obstacles.

It is important to keep in mind that legal and ethical issues are more than just boxes to be checked in this endeavour. These serve as the foundation for the patient-centered care structure. Taking care of these foundations is like taking care of a powerful tree's roots—it guarantees the tree's resilience and strength in the face of difficulty.

Thus, let's embrace the intricacies as we set out on this journey with open minds and hearts, understanding that the moral compass we carry directs not only our clinical judgments but also the fundamentals of compassionate care. By doing this, we pay respect to the distinct stories of people dealing with CHF and create a care system that is as robust and distinct as each patient we treat.

We'll go more deeply into the use of patient advocacy, ethical decision-making, and advance care planning in the context of managing chronic heart failure as we continue our investigation. Let's travel this path together, respecting each person's individuality, rights, and dignity as they negotiate the challenges of congestive heart failure.

Patient Empowerment and Self-Advocacy

My dearest warriors of the heart, it is becoming increasingly evident as we navigate the complex terrain of congestive heart failure management that patient empowerment and self-advocacy play a crucial part in ensuring our collective well-being. This chapter will examine the significant influence that taking an active role in our own care can have on the results of our health. Together, we will discover the tactics and resources that enable us to take on the role of advocates for our own health, enabling us to successfully negotiate the healthcare system with resilience and self-assurance.

In the field of managing congestive heart failure, it is critical to acknowledge the transforming power of patient empowerment and self-advocacy as we stand at the intersection of contemporary medicine and holistic wellbeing. The traditional relationship between the patient and the provider is changing, opening the door to a collaborative approach in which patients actively participate in their care, make educated decisions, and influence positive changes in their health trajectory.

The main problem is that many people with congestive heart failure have historically been given a passive role in their healthcare journey. We frequently find ourselves powerless to influence the course of our own care, carried away by the tide of medical decisions. Disempowerment, disengagement, and a sense of separation from the very processes that shape our well-being can result from this lack of agency.

This passive strategy has significant and wide-ranging repercussions. We run the risk of becoming passive characters in our own health storey if we don't actively participate in our treatment, leaving us open to choices that might not perfectly suit our own needs and goals. This mismatch can lead to less than ideal treatment results, heightened worry, and a feeling of powerlessness that compromises our general wellbeing.

The ability of patient empowerment and self-advocacy to improve lives holds the key to the solution. We reclaim our agency, voice, and power in determining the course of our health by accepting our responsibility as active participants in our care. This mentality change gives us the ability to work with our healthcare team as equal partners on our path to wellbeing, communicate our needs clearly, and make well-informed decisions.

We must first get a thorough awareness of our illness and available treatments before we can implement this approach. Equipped with this knowledge, we may ask questions, get explanation, and actively participate in collaborative decision-making in an honest and open manner with our healthcare team. Furthermore, accepting self-care routines, following treatment programmes, and speaking out for our needs reaffirm our position as proactive contributors to our own care.

There is no doubt about the evidence: people who actively participate in their own treatment have better health outcomes, a higher quality of life, and a profound sense of empowerment. By assuming responsibility for our health, we not only improve our own wellbeing but also encourage others to accept their own agency in healthcare, creating a positive feedback loop.

There isn't a one-size-fits-all strategy, my fellow heart warriors, as we traverse the waters of patient empowerment and self-advocacy. Every one of us contributes a different set of experiences, principles, and goals that help to shape our own journeys toward empowerment. The path may be difficult and confusing at times, but the benefits are immense, giving us a strong sense of resilience, purpose, and control over the storey of our health.

Alternative solutions are important in influencing the state of healthcare, even though the road of patient empowerment and self-advocacy is unquestionably revolutionary. By including peer mentoring, wellness coaching, and patient support groups, we may further increase our sense of empowerment and create a network of people who share our experiences, wisdom, and support.

My fellow heart warriors, as we come to the end of this investigation of patient empowerment and self-advocacy, I implore you to accept your responsibility as designers of your own health destiny. As a symbol of strength and fortitude, raise your voice, speak your mind, and stand tall. Let's take this transformative journey together, reshaping the healthcare environment so that patient empowerment becomes a lived reality rather than just a theoretical idea and enables us to survive in the face of hardship.

With unwavering grace and tenacity,

Dr. Ankita Kashyap

Holistic Approaches to CHF Management

Herbal Remedies and Supplements

Greetings, my dear reader, and welcome to the chapter that explores the intriguing world of nutritional supplements and herbal therapies for the treatment of congestive heart failure. As we progress toward total heart failure management, we enter the field of holistic healthcare, where the abundance of nature and the knowledge of science come together to provide a wide range of options for maintaining heart health and general well-being. So let's begin this fascinating journey toward optimal health, where traditional wisdom and cutting-edge research collide.

Imagine a tranquil setting with lush vegetation and soft sunlight kissing the ground. This is the realm of herbal cures, where the calming influence of the natural world blends with the fast-paced beat of contemporary life to provide a variety of organic remedies that promote wellbeing.

The herbal treatments and nutritional supplements that have captured the interest of wellness seekers for millennia serve as the main characters in this engrossing storey. These organic wonders, derived from minerals, herbs, and plants, have the power to support traditional medical interventions and advance heart health.

Seeking safe and efficient ways to maintain heart function and general wellness becomes difficult as we traverse the complexity of congestive heart failure. Within this complex dance between conventional and alternative medicine, the question of whether dietary supplements and herbal therapies may make a significant difference in the treatment of congestive heart failure emerges.

Here, in the spirit of holistic medicine, we unearth the particular tactics and approaches that capitalise on the potential of nutritional supplements and herbal medicines to meet the diverse needs of people with congestive heart failure. Our goal is to include these natural wonders into a comprehensive approach to heart health by gaining a thorough understanding of their properties and interactions.

We investigate a variety of nutritional supplements and herbal therapies as we go across this terrain, each having a distinct ability to promote cardiovascular health. Hawthorn's calming embrace and coenzyme Q10's energising qualities are just two of these natural partners that provide our hearts with a wide range of support. We also explore the role that heart-healthy omega-3 fatty acids play, as well as the possible advantages of specific vitamin and mineral combinations for enhancing general health.

The results of using nutritional supplements and herbal medicines in the treatment of congestive heart failure are astounding. Those who embark on this life-changing adventure may experience improved heart function, an improvement in quality of life, and a revitalization of vitality as we observe the harmonic interaction between nature's gifts and contemporary healthcare.

However, it's important to recognise that the world of nutritional supplements and herbal therapies is not without its intricacies as we make our way through it. It is imperative that we approach these natural wonders with knowledge, taking into account factors such as safety, effectiveness, and possible combinations with traditional treatments. We can safely and prudently manage these challenges by promoting a constructive conversation between traditional and modern healthcare, assuring the safe and effective integration of dietary supplements and herbal medicines into our comprehensive approach to heart health.

Visualize a visual tapestry that depicts the colourful herbs, nutritious supplements, and complex molecular dance that underlie all of the amazing natural beauties we have experienced along the way. These illustrations testify to the abundance of natural resources and their capacity to promote human well-being.

We understand the deep connection between all facets of our health as we incorporate nutritional supplements and herbal medicines into our holistic approach to heart health. The use of natural remedies in our management of Congestive Heart Failure is a reflection of the age-old maxim that health is a harmonious tapestry in which each individual component is essential to the overall harmony of well-being.

While we consider the complex dance between tradition and modernity in the field of heart health, let us consider the significant potential that dietary supplements and herbal therapies have to augment traditional treatments. How can we prudently and wisely negotiate this synergy, using nature's gifts to improve our path toward total heart failure management?

We've barely begun to explore the vast array of dietary supplements and herbal therapies that can promote heart health and general well-being in this engrossing subchapter. We'll discover the age-old knowledge and cutting-edge scientific discoveries that illuminate the way toward comprehensive management of congestive heart failure as we continue our investigation. So, dear reader, let us continue our trip toward a future in which our well-being grows in balance with nature and our hearts beat with vitality, led by the wisdom of nature and the wonders of modern science.

Acupuncture and Traditional Chinese Medicine

Treasures that have endured the test of time, enduring throughout cultures and centuries, are encountered as we travel through the many pathways of holistic healthcare and wellbeing. A combination of acupuncture and traditional Chinese medicine (TCM) offers a kaleidoscope of healing methods that balance the body, mind, and spirit, making it a promising treatment option for congestive heart failure (CHF).

Imagine a calm treatment room where the faint sound of flickering candles creates a calming atmosphere, and the air is filled with the subtle scent of burning incense. This is a haven in the middle of a busy metropolis where people who are suffering with CHF can find comfort in the age-old knowledge of TCM and acupuncture.

Enter the realm of holistic medicine, where the main characters are caring healers and keepers of age-old wisdom rather than just practitioners. Patients with CHF are seen as partners in the pursuit of vitality and balance rather than as passive beneficiaries of care in this domain. In this context, I, Dr. Ankita Kashyap, along with my team of specialists from various health and wellness domains, serve as guardians of an integrative healthcare approach that includes dietary and lifestyle adjustments, counselling and psychology-related techniques, self-help methods, alternative and complementary self-care techniques, and coping mechanisms.

The complex nature of CHF poses an enormous difficulty in the field of managing this ailment. Even though they are invaluable, conventional medical procedures frequently fall short of meeting patients' complete needs. A more holistic approach that goes beyond the confines of traditional medicine is necessary due to the subtle impacts of stress and anxiety as well as the intricate interactions between physical, emotional, and spiritual well-being.

This is the point at which the age-old understanding of TCM and acupuncture reveals its subtle but profound effectiveness. Acupuncture aims to restore the body's natural flow of vital energy, or Qi, via a delicate dance of needles. By carefully positioning these tiny needles, symptoms are reduced and a feeling of wellbeing is promoted as the body is gently pushed toward equilibrium. With its complex formulas, traditional Chinese herbal medicine provides a gentle yet effective ally in bringing the body's systems back into balance. When combined with traditional therapies, these modalities create a potent therapeutic mosaic that attends to patients' emotional and psychological struggles in addition to their physical CHF symptoms.

The results of using TCM and acupuncture together in the treatment of CHF are astounding. Along with a decrease in bodily symptoms like edoema and dyspnea, patients often report feeling more resilient and alive. Additionally, a significant change in the emotional and psychological terrain is brought about by the holistic approach, enabling patients to face the difficulties of CHF with renewed grace and resilience. The evidence is overwhelming, as studies show that including acupuncture and TCM into the treatment of congestive heart failure improves cardiac function, quality of life, and lowers hospitalisation rates.

We are forced to marvel at the great knowledge contained within these age-old healing therapies when we look upon the tapestry weaved by acupuncture and TCM in the context of managing CHF. However, we must also be aware of the subtleties and possible objections that may surface in our reverence. In order to bridge the gap between conventional wisdom and scientifically supported medicine, the combination of acupuncture and TCM necessitates a careful tango between tradition and technology. Even while the results speak for themselves, we still need to exercise caution when traversing this territory to make sure patients get the best of both worlds without sacrificing efficacy or safety.

Imagine a picture of the complex meridians and acupoints that are the basis of acupuncture, like rivers and tributaries that flow across the body's topography, enhancing and balancing it. Consider the delicate equilibrium between yin and yang, the basic principles of traditional Chinese medicine, as a metaphor for the equilibrium that CHF management aims to achieve.

The use of TCM and acupuncture into the management of congestive heart failure goes beyond simple treatment; it represents a revolution in healthcare. It calls us to honour the complex interactions between mind, body, and spirit and to embrace the wisdom of old traditions and incorporate them into contemporary medicine. It alludes to a broader storey of holistic well-being in which the search for vitality and balance serves as the cornerstone of healthcare and extends beyond the boundaries of specific illnesses to encompass the full range of human experience.

Let us consider the timeless wisdom contained in these age-old methods as we consider the significant implications of incorporating TCM and acupuncture into the management of CHF. In order to acknowledge the healing fabric that crosses generations and cultures, how may we continue to bridge the gaps between tradition and contemporary in healthcare? What new avenues for health and wellbeing may we explore in this tango between the old and the new? Come along with me as we continue to explore the complex web of holistic health and wellness, informed by both the limitless possibilities of modern medicine and the wisdom of ancient traditions.

Ayurveda and Holistic Wellness

Greetings, reader, from a world where the traditional knowledge of Ayurveda and the contemporary philosophy of holistic health join together to change the treatment of congestive heart failure. Accompany me on an exploration that goes beyond conventional medical frameworks and explores the interrelated domains of customised lifestyle approaches, food guidance, and the equilibrium between mind and body.

Imagine a busy clinic where the soft hum of healing energy blends with the aroma of calming essential oils. Patients are treated as persons in this setting, with distinct histories, motivations, and stories—not just names on a chart. The values of Ayurveda and holistic wellbeing, which embrace the full person rather than just treating the symptoms, come to life in this caring setting.

I am honoured to collaborate with a group of professionals from many health and wellness domains in this all-encompassing strategy for controlling congestive heart failure. Together, we construct a tapestry of knowledge, experience, and compassion, weaving together the threads of traditional and modern therapeutic approaches. Not only do we aim to relieve symptoms, but we also want to provide our patients the tools they need to live healthy, active lives.

Congestive heart failure is a difficult condition that affects people's emotional and spiritual health in addition to their physical health. Conventional medical treatments frequently ignore the holistic part of the human experience in favour of only treating the physiological aspects of the illness. Patients may feel disengaged from their own healing process as a result of this limited approach and long for a more all-encompassing answer.

Let us introduce you to Ayurveda, the traditional Indian medical system that treats every person as a distinct combination of the elements. We customise our treatment for each patient using the principles of Ayurveda, taking into account their lifestyle, mental health, and dosha constitution. Customized diet plans include heart-healthy foods and herbs that support heart health and harmonise with the body's natural rhythms.

However, our strategy goes beyond the dish. We explore the area of mind-body balance, incorporating yoga, meditation, and customised lifestyle techniques to foster inner peace and emotional resiliency. Our patients are more than just people in need of medical attention; they are engaged agents in their own recovery, equipped with the knowledge and ability to make decisions that are relevant to their particular circumstances.

This all-encompassing strategy produces results that are truly revolutionary. Patients report a significant improvement in their general state of well-being in addition to a decrease in their physical problems. They report better mood, more vitality, and an overall sense of empowerment that goes beyond their diagnosis. These findings are corroborated by data, which shows quantifiable gains in heart function, decreased inflammation, and improved quality of life.

When we consider these results, it is clear that managing congestive heart failure holistically has several advantages that go well beyond the scope of traditional medical treatments. We respect the interdependence of body, mind, and spirit by adopting the principles of Ayurveda and holistic wellness, realising that genuine healing embraces all facets of the human experience.

Imagine a colourful mandala that embodies this holistic approach, combining mindfulness, movement, spirituality, and nutrition to create a healing symphony. Every component is linked with the others to create a harmonious picture of wellbeing that goes beyond the bounds of conventional medical paradigms.

Ayurveda and holistic health care are not separate endeavours when it comes to managing congestive heart failure. It represents a wider storey of change in the field of healthcare—a move away from reductionist methods and toward a broader, more inclusive healing paradigm. It challenges us to reevaluate how we view health and wellness and to embrace the significant role that individualised, all-encompassing treatments play in the treatment of long-term illnesses.

During our exploration of Ayurveda and holistic wellness, I would like you to consider this: Could it be that the future of healthcare does not lie in isolated treatments but rather in the fusion of traditional knowledge with contemporary science, creating a healing fabric that values the whole person?

We will go deeper into the concepts of Ayurveda and holistic wellness in the pages that follow. We will examine the complex dance of dietary guidelines, mind-body balance, and customised lifestyle routines in the context of managing congestive heart failure. Together, let's set out on a journey of exploration as we embrace the life-changing possibilities of a holistic approach to wellbeing.

Energy Healing and Reiki

It's hard to ignore the significant influence of energy healing modalities like Reiki as we dive deeper into the complex realm of holistic healthcare and wellbeing. Imagine the following: a calm space filled with ambient light that is soft and pervasive, a soft bubbling fountain, and a subtle hint of lavender remaining in the air. It is in this tranquil environment that we find people battling the complications of congestive heart failure and looking for relief and recovery via complementary and alternative methods.

Within this field of healing, we come across a wide range of participants: people who are experiencing Congestive Heart Failure and the professionals who help them achieve emotional stability and calm. Our investigation takes place against a backdrop of hope and resiliency, with each participant attempting to meet the obstacles this condition presents with dignity and resolve.

The central problem of our storey is the complex network of psychological and physical suffering that frequently coexists with congestive heart failure. With its taxing symptoms and the constant fear of death, this illness can have a profound emotional impact on people who are afflicted. We are forced to look for holistic treatments that nurture the spirit just as much as they heal the body because we must address the illness's emotional effects in addition to its physical symptoms.

Step in Reiki and energy healing, which shine through the storm like rays of hope. These techniques provide a distinct method for helping people navigating the complex landscape of congestive heart failure to relax, reduce tension, and improve their emotional well-being. The methodology is based on the knowledge that genuine healing must take care of all three aspects of the human experience, which are woven together into a tapestry.

Along the way, we see firsthand the transforming impact of these practises as people find relief from the turmoil caused by their disease. Reiki practitioners help their clients reestablish a connection with the inherent harmony of their being by creating a space for restoration through the gentle laying on of hands and the channelling of universal life force energy. Those who use these modalities report significant and far-reaching benefits in their emotional stability, a general sense of serenity and well-being, and lower stress levels.

Thinking back on this case study, we are struck by how amazing it is that the human spirit can heal and regenerate itself, even in the face of overwhelming adversity. The outcomes are very telling, presenting a picture of resiliency and rejuvenation that goes beyond the purview of traditional medicine. The visual aids that accompany this inquiry provide a window into the subtle yet profound alterations that take place inside the domain of the heart and soul, and serve as poignant reminders of the transformational power of energy healing.

By relating this storey to the broader healthcare system, we are reminded of how crucial it is to adopt a holistic approach to recovery. With elegance and grace, the interdependent relationship between the material and the immaterial, the physical and the metaphysical, is emphasised, challenging us to broaden our conception of health and well-being. What if we accepted the idea that true healing includes not just the healing of the body but also the upholding of the spirit and the comforting of the soul? This question remains in the air, like the faint echo of a melody?

Thus, we are standing at the cusp of opportunity, staring into the infinite horizon of holistic health and wellness. The journey that takes place is one of regeneration and discovery, challenging our preconceived notions of health and well-being. Let us bring with us the knowledge of the past and the hope of a future filled with empathy and comprehension as we set out on our journey, for it is only through the combination of these factors that congestive heart failure may be truly conquered.

Mindfulness and Meditation

Greetings from the path of holistic health and total well-being, dear reader. It gives me great joy to introduce you to the life-changing potential of mindfulness and meditation as we set out on this adventure together. For people navigating the complications of congestive heart failure, these age-old practices—often disregarded in the field of contemporary medicine—hold the key to opening up a world of inner serenity, emotional resilience, and physical vigour.

Let's start by discussing the fundamentals of mindfulness and meditation. The practise of mindfulness involves focusing entirely on the present moment and letting go of judgement and attachment to the past or future. It is the peaceful practise of compassionately observing our thoughts, feelings, and physical sensations. By doing this, we can develop a profound sense of inner clarity and tranquilly. However, the deliberate practise of stilling the mind and turning our attention inward—usually through breathwork, visualisation, or guided contemplation—is known as meditation. When combined, these techniques create a harmonic whole that leads us to a deep sense of peace and self-awareness.

The fundamental principles of mindfulness and meditation come from the age-old knowledge of Eastern traditions, where sages and seekers of enlightenment attempted to solve the enigmas surrounding the human mind and soul. The roots of the idea of mindfulness may be found in Buddhist teachings, where it was considered the primary means of achieving enlightenment and mental development. Similar to this, meditation has been a crucial component of many spiritual traditions, offering a route to self-realization and transcendence. These traditional methods have become a part of contemporary healthcare, providing a comprehensive approach to recovery that goes beyond the purview of traditional medicine.

Let's now discuss the significant benefits of mindfulness and meditation in the context of managing congestive heart failure. Imagine the heart as the literal and figurative centre of our existence. Its vitality is closely related to our general well-being, and its rhythm reflects the ebb and flow of our emotions. The burden of managing congestive heart failure can frequently result in increased stress, worry, and emotional instability for those who have it. This is where meditation and mindfulness become vital partners, providing a haven of peace amidst the chaos of changing lifestyles and medical complications.

Think about the turbulent emotional waves that frequently follow a congestive heart failure diagnosis. The very condition we are trying to control might be made worse by feelings of fear, uncertainty, and frustration. People can learn to accept their feelings with compassionate awareness and face their concerns head-on by engaging in the peaceful practise of mindfulness. Through practising an accepting and uncritical presence in the here and now, we can unravel the maze of worry and discover comfort in the basic act of breathing and existing.

Furthermore, it is impossible to overestimate the physiological advantages of mindfulness and meditation. These techniques have been demonstrated in studies to lower blood pressure, lessen inflammation, and enhance heart health in general. By incorporating these techniques into our daily lives, we can establish a mental retreat where our hearts beat in time with the tranquil beat of our inner selves.

The practical uses of mindfulness and meditation in the treatment of congestive heart failure are virtually endless. Imagine a patient who finds comfort in some quiet time each day to ponder after a long day of doctor's appointments and drug schedules. They get the resilience and grace necessary to manage the intricacies of their situation under the kind supervision of mindfulness. Imagine another person, facing the psychological effects of congestive heart failure, learning about the transformative potential of meditation as they set out on a path of self-awareness and emotional equilibrium.

However, despite the many advantages of mindfulness and meditation, there are several widespread myths that can obscure their actual benefits. Some people might write these activities off as mere esoteric pleasures, but they have real health benefits and are supported by science. Some people might think that practising mindfulness and meditation takes hours upon hours of laborious effort, not realising that even a short period of focused thought can have profound effects. It is imperative to debunk these myths and accept these practises as approachable methods of nourishing the body, mind, and spirit.

Let us not undervalue the significant benefits of mindfulness and meditation as we make our way through the maze of congestive heart failure treatment. A path to comprehensive healing, a haven of peace, and a ray of hope can all be found in the soft embrace of these age-old traditions. Let's take this transforming journey together, learning to cultivate an inner calm and attentive presence that goes beyond disease and adversity. Discover a tranquil world within by allowing mindfulness and meditation to heal your heart.

We will explore the use of mindfulness and meditation to the treatment of congestive heart failure in more detail in the pages that follow, including useful techniques and touching case studies that demonstrate their transformational power. Come along with me as we set off on this healing journey, honouring the timeless knowledge and the unbreakable spirit of humanity. Together, let's open the door to comprehensive congestive heart failure care by learning the profound art of meditation and unlocking the secrets of mindful living.

Aromatherapy and Relaxation Techniques

Greetings, my dear reader, from a place where the art of relaxation and the power of aroma combine to create a haven for tired souls. We shall travel through the healing powers of aromatherapy and relaxation techniques in this subchapter, revealing their significant influence on the treatment of congestive heart failure. Imagine this: a peaceful environment with soft lighting casting a gentle glow, comforting essential oil scents dancing through the air, and a mental escape from the hectic pace of everyday life. We will explore the transforming power of these practises here, in this sanctuary of holistic healing, recognising their capacity to nourish the body as well as the spirit.

Let me introduce you to the main characters as we enter this world of wellness: the historical and highly esteemed ancient art of relaxation, as well as the aromatic essences extracted from nature's abundance. These are the instruments we will use to help folks who are suffering from congestive heart failure by providing comfort and assistance.

Congestive heart failure is a serious condition that affects a lot of people, making it a difficult struggle to overcome. A feeling of anxiety and restlessness might be brought on by the heart's unwavering rhythm, which is reduced by the severity of this ailment. By creating a healthy balance between the body and the mind, we aim to provide solace and respite in this vulnerable region.

Our strategy is to embrace the healing properties of aromatherapy and relaxation techniques while providing gentle instruction and unshakable support. Our goal is to create a sense of quiet and tranquillity by calming the turbulent waters of the heart with a skillful blend of essential oils, each of which has special healing qualities. When incorporated into daily life, these techniques support the person on their path to holistic wellbeing by acting as resilient threads.

Let us now focus on the outcomes of our efforts, as this is where the real magic happens. When aromatherapy and relaxation techniques are used, congestive heart failure patients have reported a noticeable improvement in their overall health. Calming and calming effects have been facilitated by the calming influence of frankincense, the energising effect of peppermint, and the soft hug of lavender. After bearing the weight of its hardships for a while, the heart finds a moment of release and begins to dance to the tune of tranquilly and harmony.

A deep fact becomes apparent when we take time to examine and consider these results: the healing power of nature transcends the boundaries of traditional medicine. It is found in the deft application of a calming aroma, the soft assurance of peace, and the graceful flow of relaxation. The experiences of those who have adopted these techniques attest to their significant influence, even though some may doubt their effectiveness.

Visual aids become our companions in this investigation, providing a window into the realm of relaxation and aromatherapy. Imagine the gentle swirls of fragrant mist, the vivid colours of essential oils, and the peaceful scenes that invite the tired spirit to take a break. The reader is invited to enter a world where the senses are awakened and the spirit finds comfort through these visuals, which act as windows into a healing realm.

When we relate these experiences to the broader storey of managing congestive heart failure, we find a basic reality: there are a plethora of options on the way to healing. It grows on the rich soil of holistic techniques rather than being restricted to the stiff frameworks of traditional medicine. When approached with an open mind and an inquisitive heart, aromatherapy and relaxation techniques become allies in the pursuit of comprehensive well-being.

And with that, my dear reader, I leave you with this notion to consider: where may you find a moment of peace and relief in the middle of life's chaos? Maybe it lingers in the soft whisper of a scented breeze, or in the silent hug of a peaceful place. Let's look for these times of relaxation as we travel together, knowing that they can contain healing seeds ready to sprout.

We will continue to examine the various routes to wellness that lie ahead as we delve deeper into the holistic care of congestive heart failure in the pages that follow. Until then, may the elegant dance of relaxation and the soft murmurs of essential oils lead you on your path to a peaceful heart.

Integrative Medicine and Collaborative Care

Greetings, my dear reader, from a world where complementary and alternative therapies beat in perfect harmony with the pulse of orthodox medicine. At the core of our strategy for treating congestive heart failure is a belief that treats the patient as a whole, not just the illness. Let me give you a clear picture of our collaborative care model and the transformative potential it possesses as we set out on this adventure.

Envision a busy medical facility where the aura of optimism and healing permeates every corner. This is no typical clinic—rather, it's a haven where a variety of professionals come together to share their individual specialties and weave a tapestry of health. Here, the sterile tang of medical equipment blends with the aroma of calming herbs, signifying the union of traditional knowledge and cutting-edge science.

As a physician and health and wellness coach, I lead this symphony of care, passionately promoting holistic health that verges on poetry. Beside me, a group of professionals from other fields makes up the foundation of our integrative methodology. We have experts in nutrition, acupuncture, psychology, yoga, and other fields, and they all bring their unique skills to the table.

The intricate network of difficulties that congestive heart failure presents is the central theme of our storey. Millions of lives are affected by this disorder, which is defined by the heart's incapacity to pump blood efficiently. Despite their importance, conventional treatments frequently fail to adequately address the disease's complex nature. Patients struggle with emotional, mental, and spiritual distress in addition to physical symptoms, necessitating a more all-encompassing approach.

Then along comes integrative medicine, a ray of hope amidst the chronic illness storm. Our strategy aims to enhance traditional therapies by including alternative modalities into the overall care plan, rather than to replace them. For example, we create custom meal programmes, offer lifestyle counselling, and research psychology to identify coping mechanisms that enable patients to successfully negotiate the psychological maze associated with their illness.

We also welcome complementary therapies like yoga, acupuncture, and mindfulness exercises, understanding their ability to lighten the load of symptoms and calm the soul. By fostering the mind-body connection, we help our patients develop a strong sense of resilience and provide them with a powerful toolkit to combat the challenges associated with congestive heart failure.

Our hard work has concrete results that have a profound impact; the results are not just abstract concepts. Our patients, who had previously accepted the limitations of their illness, now feel empowered by their renewed energy. They talk about better sleep, less stress and anxiety, and a sense of empowerment that goes beyond being sick. Furthermore, objective metrics demonstrate improved heart function and a decrease in readmissions to the hospital, highlighting the effectiveness of our strategy.

I'm struck, when I look back on our journey, by the deep lessons woven throughout our collaborative care paradigm. Of course, there are difficulties and detractors of it. Some sceptics might doubt the scientific foundation of some complementary therapies, while others would express worries about the possibility of receiving contradictory advice from different professionals. These are chances for discussion and improvement rather than insurmountable challenges.

Our integrative approach reminds us that the human experience transcends reductionism in the big theatre of healthcare. It calls us to acknowledge the wonderful complexity of every person and the fact that healing is more than just filling out a prescription pad. Our experience invites us to see health through a kaleidoscope lens that refracts the light of other disciplines, demonstrating the transforming power of holistic care.

Envision a graph that represents the course of a patient's health, with the ascending line representing the rise in hope and energy following integrative care. Imagine a mandala; its complex designs represent the unity of the mind, body, and spirit, serving as a visual representation of our therapeutic method.

Our storey of integrative medicine and teamwork in healthcare is not a stand-alone vignette, but rather a microcosm of a greater storey that honours the union of innovation and tradition, science and art, in the service of human happiness. It invites us to reconsider healthcare as a patchwork of varied perspectives, each adding a crucial shade to the healing canvas.

As we make our way through the maze of managing congestive heart failure, consider this: What if there was no distinction between conventional and complementary medicines, creating a smooth continuum of care? In what ways could this paradigm change benefit the lives of both practitioners and patients? Accompany me as we explore the field of integrative medicine and address these questions, using knowledge as our guide and compassion as our compass.

Printed in the USA
CPSIA information can be obtained
at www.ICGtesting.com
LVHW011021311223
767822LV00017BA/1813

9 798215 552001